Sheila Kitzinger

REDISCOVERING BIRTH

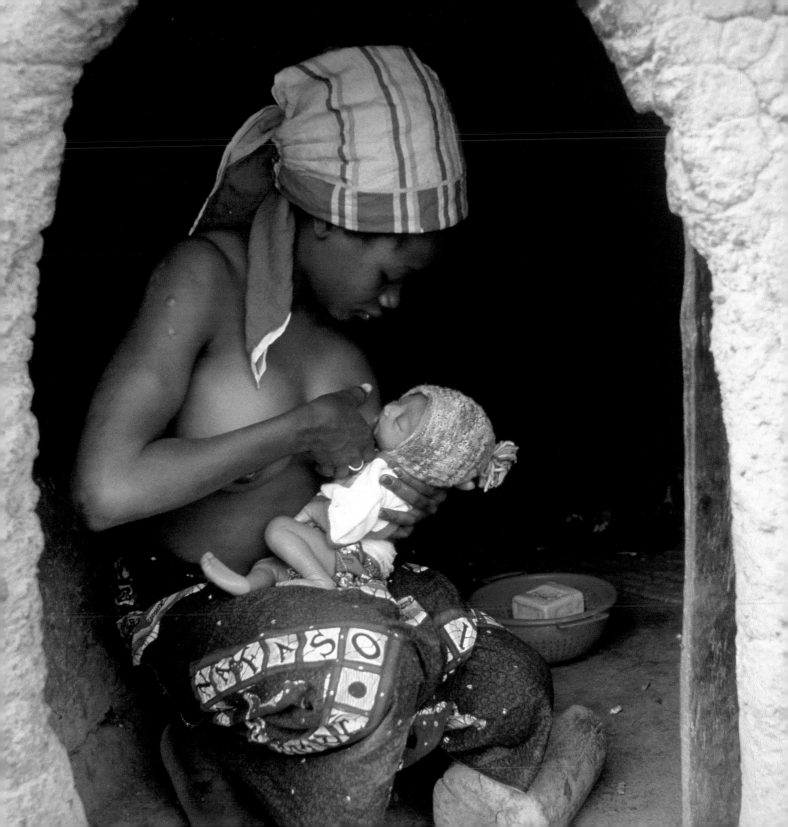

Sheila Kitzinger

REDISCOVERING BIRTH

LITTLE, BROWN

BOSTON · NEW YORK · LONDON

A Little, Brown Book

First published in 2000 by Little, Brown and Company (UK).

Text by Sheila Kitzinger © copyright 2000.

The moral right of the author has been asserted.

A CIP catalogue record for this book is available from the
British Library.

ISBN 0-316-85393-3

Designed by Janet James

Little, Brown and Company (UK)
Brettenham House, Lancaster Place,
London WC2E 7EN

Page 2 Mark Edwards/Still Pictures; Page 5 Sheila Kitzinger; Page 7 J. Kitzinger; Page 13 Mark Hakansson/Panos Pictures; Page 15 Ann Shamel G.; Page 16 Sean Sprague/Panos Pictures; Page 17 Museum for Textiles, Toronto; Page 18 Robyn Kahukiwa/Roma Potiki; Page 21 Marcia May; Page 22 Eva Zielinska-Millar, The Royal Collection; Page 23 Wellcome Library, London; Page 24 (left) Yale University, Harvey Cushing/John Hay Whitney Medical Library, Historical Collection; Page 24 (right) National Library of Medicine; Page 25 National Library of Medicine; Page 26 (left) The Bridgeman Art Library; Page 26 (right) M. Ravenna, Museo di Anatomia Umana, Bologna; Page 27 National Library of Medicine, Bethesda, Md.; Page 29 Images Colour Library; Page 30 Sandra Lousada; Page 35 Joe Partridge; Page 39 Tony Latham, Tony Stone Images; Page 41 Masako Miyazaki; Page 43 (left) Sheila Kitzinger; Page 43 (right) The Bridgeman Art Library; Page 47 Laura Cao-Romero; Page 51 Guadalupe Trueba; Page 54 John Loy/MIDIRS photo library; Page 56 Neil Cooper/Panos Pictures; Page 59 Venezia Biblioteca Querini Stampalia; Page 60 *A History of Childbirth in America*, Richard W. Wertz and Dorothy C. Wertz; Page 61 (left) Advertising Archives; Page 61 (right) John Stilwell/PA News Photo Library; Page 65 Rex Features; Page 67 Durgha Bernhard; Page 68 G. Helmes; Page 70 (top) AKG London/Erich Lessing; Page 70 (bottom) e.t.archive; Page 71 (background) Museum for Textiles, Toronto; Page 71 (inset) Joe Partridge; Page 72 Joe Partridge; Page 75 National Museum, Athens; Page 76 The Louvre, Paris; Page 77 e.t.archive; Page 78 AKG London/Erich Lessing; Page 79 (top) Leiden Museum, Netherlands; Page 79 (bottom) AKG London/Erich Lessing; Page 80 (top) Marija Gimbutas; Page 80 (bottom) Sheila Kitzinger; Page 81 AKG London/Erich Lessing; Page 82 Joe Partridge; Page 83 Joe Partridge; Page 89 The Huntington Library, California; Page 91 'Born in the USA', Patchworks Productions 2000; Page 92 Crispin Hughes/Panos Pictures; Page 95 Giacomo Pirozzi/Panos Pictures; Page 97 AKG London; Page 98 AKG London/Erich Lessing; Page 100 *Childbirth and Authoritative Knowledge* by Robbie E. Davis-Floyd and Carolyn F. Sargent; Page 106 Bibloteque Nationale, Paris; Page 107 (left) Museo de Arte de Cataluna (Barcelona); Page 115 Wellcome Library, London; Page 121 Museum Boijmans Van Beuningen; Page 124 Sue Gerber; Page 125 Steven Robert Coleman/Panos Pictures; Page 129 Bubbles/Gena Naccache; Page 130 The British Library; Page 133 Bodleian Library; Page 134 Sharon Blackmon; Page 137 Jack Delano, Library of Congress Prints; Page 143 'Born in the USA', Patchworks Productions 2000; Page 144 Giacomo Pirozzi/Panos Pictures; Pages 148-9 Nancy Durrell McKenna; Page 155 Andre Maslennikov/Still Pictures; Page 165 Marcia May; Page 167 Sheila Kitzinger; Page 168 Marcia May; Page 169 (right) Nancy Durrell McKenna; Pages 170-1 Margaret Mead; Page 174 Eve Arnold/Magnum Photos; Page 176 Joe Partridge; Page 178 Dave Saunders; Page 179 Fanny Di Cara; Page 181 Marcia May; Page 183 Sally Greenhill; Page 184 Marcia May; Page 187-8 Dave Saunders; Page 189 Joe Partridge; Pages 190-1 Dave Saunders; Page 192 (top) Dave Saunders; Page 192 (bottom left) National Museum of Science and Industry, London; Page 193 (top) Nancy Durrell McKenna; Page 193 (bottom) industrie malvestio guido s.p.a.; Page 194 Marcia May; Page 197 Marcia May; Page 199 Hattie Young/Science Photo Library; Page 200 Yasuko Funamoto; Page 203 *Obstetrics for Nurses* by Joseph DeLee; Page 205 E. Duigenan-Christian Aid/Still Pictures; Page 207 Guadalupe Trueba; Page 208 Joe Partridge; Page 209 Bill Stephenson/Panos Pictures; Page 211 Dave Saunders; Page 214 'Born in the USA', Patchworks Productions 2000; Page 217 Victoria Smith/SOA; Page 218 Liba Taylor/Panos Pictures; Page 220 Dean Chapman/Panos Pictures; Page 223 Sean Ellis, Tony Stone Images; Page 231 Mark Hakansson/Panos Pictures; Page 234 Guadalupe Trueba; Page 235 TCL Stock Directory; Page 237 Mark Edwards/Still Pictures; Page 238 Ms Ines Avellana-Fernandez; Page 245 Giacomo Pirozzi/Panos Pictures

Every effort has been made to trace the copyright holders of the illustrative material included in this book, but if any have been inadvertently overlooked the publishers will be pleased to make the necessary arrangement at the first opportunity.

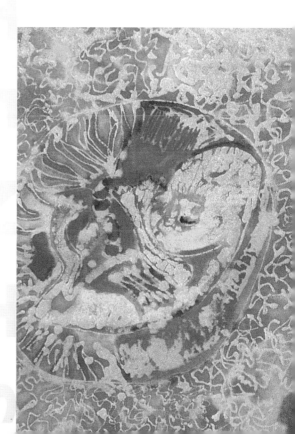

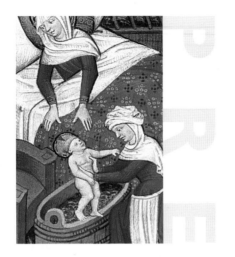

This book is the outcome of birth research and discussion with midwives, mothers, doctors and sociologists in many different countries. It has been a rich experience for me to sit with women in labour in countries as far apart as Italy, Russia, Mexico, Poland, Japan, South Africa, Britain, Iceland, France, the Czech Republic, Australia, Germany and Hungary, and I want to thank all those who have given me the opportunity to do this and have made me so welcome. Wherever possible I have provided references for the material used. Where no references are given, the material comes from my own field research in different cultures.

I should like to thank the Medical Research Council Unit at the University of the West Indies in Jamaica which generously provided the base for my original research in the 1960s. Agathe Scamporrino and the midwives in Palermo, Sakae Kikuchi and Ritsuko Toda in Japan, Gabrielle Palmer and Mr Feng in China, Beatrijs Smulders in Holland, particularly for the information she has given me about birth in Bali, Melanie Habanananda in Thailand, Laura Cao-Romero and Guadalupe Trueba in Mexico, Janet Ashford in the United States, Janet Chawla and Priya Vincent in India, and the Pauktuutit Inuit Women's Association of Canada have all helped me a great deal. Thank you also to the many midwives who sent me copies of historic midwifery textbooks, and to MIDIRS, the Midwives Information and Resource Service, for help with photographs. I am grateful to Mary Barnard for translating material from the Dutch. Some of the aspects of touch referred to in Chapter 7 are covered in a different form in my account of 'Authoritative Touch in Childbirth' in Robbie Davis-Floyd's and Carolyn Sargent's book *Childbirth and Authoritative Knowledge*, and academic readers would do well to study that book, too.

Stimulating discussions with my sociologist daughter Jenny Kitzinger, Lesley Page, the Queen Charlotte's Professor of Midwifery, have been helpful, and my husband, Uwe, spared the time from sailing for a critical reading of the whole manuscript, and my daughter Polly Kitzinger helped with proofreading.

The book would never have seen the light of day without enthusiastic secretarial assistance first from Jane Young, then from Rachel Clark, and finally Jennifer Darnley. And if I hadn't been able to rely on Hazel Wilce for housekeeping I would have had to spend time with a vacuum cleaner instead of a computer.

And talking of computers, my warmest thanks go to my daughter Tess who, an electronic engineer by training, for the moment a full time mother of three, has supported my work both in terms of ideas and technology, and has also designed and manages my web site: www.sheilakitzinger.com

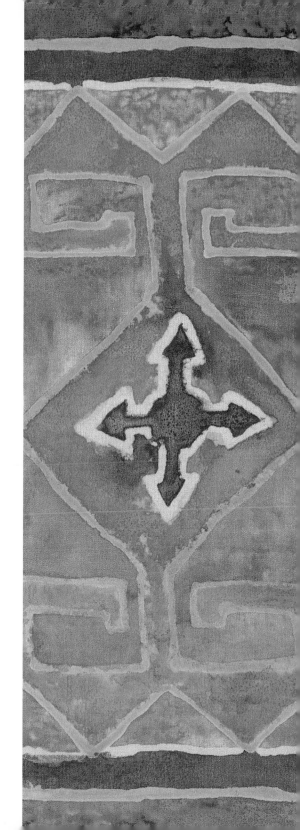

SEARCHING QUESTIONS ABOUT BIRTH

For many thousands of years, and still in certain cultures across the world, women have given birth among people they know in a place they know well, usually their own home. Knowledge is shared between the participants and the act of bringing a baby into the world is a social event.

In northern industrial societies today, when a woman gets pregnant she may be presented with various options. Yet if she is having her first baby she has only the vaguest idea of how birth really feels and how other women cope. Birth is set apart from the rest of women's lives and accepted as a matter of specialist knowledge. Because our culture of childbirth is intensely medicalised, choices are polarised: to have an epidural or manage without painkillers; to agree to electronic fetal monitoring or refuse it; to decide on a Caesarean section or to deliver vaginally; to put complete trust in the obstetrician or to summon up the courage to go it alone; to accept all the interventions that are proposed or to try for 'natural childbirth'.

But it doesn't have to be this way. To make genuine choices it helps to have a wider perspective. A woman can make use of modern obstetric skills and technology if and when she needs them. And she can explore everything that has been learned about birth through time and in different cultures so that she can labour using the shared knowledge of countless women. While acknowledging the tough lives women have in many societies, it is easy to ignore the positive aspects of traditional birth practices, and the many ways that are known of keeping birth 'normal', allowing it to unfold physiologically rather than under medical control.

In most northern industrialised cultures we have come to expect a certain kind of childbirth. It takes place in a hospital, among strangers. Pregnancy and birth are 'managed' by care-givers who assume that they know more about what is happening than the woman who is bearing the child. Her body is treated as a machine which is constantly at risk of breaking down. The safe removal of the baby from the maternal body which threatens it depends on the expertise of a group of professionals with a closed and esoteric system of knowledge. So birth is a medical, and often a surgical, event.

Each woman having a baby in hospital is transformed into a patient. She is a temporary member of a tightly organised, hierarchic and bureaucratic medical system. The admission procedure marks the point at which the institution takes control over her body.

Each woman having a baby in hospital is transformed into a patient.

It is a formal ceremony in which she is registered, classified, examined, the fetal heart rate is recorded, and her blood pressure is measured. In Eastern European countries a ceremonial cleansing is still carried out: the woman's bowels are emptied with an enema and she is reduced to a prepubertal state by having her pubic hair shaved.

In most hospitals a woman surrenders her own clothing, a symbol of her individuality, and wears the uniform provided by the institution. She is separated from friends and family, with the exception nowadays of a designated birth partner. She becomes, as it were, a child herself, expected to follow instructions, avoid drawing attention to herself and behave nicely. She may be addressed by her first name, but rarely calls the obstetricians by their first name, or she may be further de-personalised by losing her name altogether, and is referred to by professionals as 'the Caesarean in room 16', 'the pre-eclampsia case', 'the grand multip', or 'the induction'. She usually strives to be a good patient.

When interns in a Boston hospital were asked to define a 'good patient', one reply was, 'She does what I say, hears what I say, believes what I say . . .'[1] A good patient is compliant. Not only does she conform, but she thanks the professionals because they 'save' her baby. She is grateful regardless of what they do to her. Women who fail to conform in this way are seen as 'difficult patients'.

It has become normal in hospitals for birth to be regulated by artificial hormones and often completed by surgery. The woman is attended by a team of professionals. She may be tethered to electronic equipment, be numbed by anaesthesia from the waist down and have her uterus artificially stimulated. Then an episiotomy is performed and she may be delivered by forceps, vacuum extractor or ultimately a Caesarean section. Alternatively, the decision may be made to avoid labour entirely and to schedule an elective Caesarean section instead. Or the woman may request a Caesarean because she has been led to believe that this is the easiest, safest and most pain-free way to have a baby.

Every institution has rules and norms of practice; the larger the institution, the more rules there are. Every hospital has protocols so that each member of the hierarchy knows their place and there is no need to use individual initiative. Protocols are convenient, make for easy management, and enable those at a higher level to regulate the actions of

> **The culture of a society is made up of all the meanings that are so deeply inscribed into our everyday actions that we rarely question them. It is most evident in the great transitions of life: birth, puberty, marriage and death.**

their subordinates. Similarly, routines ensure that people co-operate in tasks without asking awkward questions or having to think, and as a result they are rarely challenged. When evidence-based research is published which shows that a particular custom or intervention is useless or harmful, it takes around fifteen years for it to effectively change obstetric practice.[2]

A woman who wishes to give birth as naturally as possible, prefers to have no drugs, and chooses midwife care, may be transferred to specialised obstetric care as soon as there are signs of deviation from the normal. Midwives are often anxious about the responsibility they take on when they attend out-of-hospital births, and even births in 'home-from-home' rooms in the hospital. The result is that a high percentage of women who hope to give birth without intervention are wheeled across the corridor or transported by ambulance to hi-tech care. This often happens because their membranes rupture early or labour is slow.

We live in a society where it is taken for granted that birth is a medical event which usually takes place in hospital and is thought about almost exclusively in terms of risk. Women who make the decision to give birth at home must usually overcome many obstacles put in place by the medical system. Family members and friends say, 'You're very brave!', 'Aren't you worried that something will go wrong?', and often 'You are being selfish', or 'You're not thinking about the baby'.

When birth is complicated it is safer to be in a hospital. In obstructed labour a Caesarean section can be performed, postpartum haemorrhage treated, an adherent placenta delivered, a hysterectomy done, and preterm and sick babies saved. But today straightforward labours also tend to be treated with all the interventions that are characteristic of high risk births. Treated as high risk, they often become high risk.

History and Anthropology

The culture of a society is made up of all the meanings that are so deeply inscribed into our everyday actions that we rarely question them. It is most evident in the great transitions of life: birth, puberty, marriage and death. To begin to understand the patterns of culture, and how they change and impact on each other, we have to examine the birth process in different societies across the globe, and in their and our own pasts.

Throughout this book I draw on history, social anthropology and art to better understand the challenges that face us in birth today. These are usually distinct and separate studies. The story of our past is treated quite differently from the description of other cultures, while sculpture, painting and other symbolic representations of powerful values and ways of seeing the world provide merely incidental decoration. Yet ignoring history, anthropology and art can lead to a dangerous tunnel vision. Social anthropology, for example, not only reveals how other people behave, it enables us to understand our own culture, past and present. We gain a new perspective. In the same way, art reveals layers of meaning in each culture and shocks us into a new perception.

The Victorians saw history as a mountain; thanks to Christianity, commerce and invention they were at its summit. Missionaries, travellers and ethnologists who wrote about the peculiar practices of the people they encountered in Africa, the Pacific Islands and the Far East assumed vast superiority and believed that they were able to study the social behaviour and beliefs of 'primitives' with lofty detachment. Their books recorded, often in painstaking detail, the curiosities, bizarre superstitions and grotesque ceremonies of alien cultures. Frazer's *The Golden Bough* is the best known example of this genre.

The medical model of birth is only one among many. In this book I look to history, cross-cultural anthropology, and the expression of human values through art in an attempt to understand the nature of birth in technocratic as well as in preindustrial and traditional societies.[3]

The Way We 'See' and Record Childbirth

One way of 'seeing' birth is to record it as a series of bio-medical events within a time framework: the strength and frequency of contractions, dilatation of the cervix, analgesia given, maternal blood pressure, fetal heart rate, descent and rotation of the fetal head, the management of labour and method of delivery, and so on.

Another way of 'seeing' birth is to describe the relationships between those participating: who comes and goes, the effect of their presence or absence, what they do, and what goes on in the space between the different actors. This includes jokes and laughter, expressions of emotion, and observations and information that are shared or withheld between members of the group and with the woman in labour. It entails recording any stresses evident between the various actors, and the liaisons they form, movement towards and away from each other, the use of touch – who touches, when and with what purpose, and the messages conveyed and received through touch – the body language of everyone involved, and the ritual activities enacted because they introduce an assurance of safety, simply because they are always done that way.

The first type of record is the partogram, a graph of events during childbirth. The second is the way in which a social anthropologist or social psychologist observes birth. Both ways of 'seeing' are valid. They are observations of two different levels of human behaviour. Each affects the other. In this book I look at a major life experience, shared by women all over the world and throughout time, as an anthropologist and sociologist. My focus is the relation between the psychological, the social and the physiological.

Becoming aware of the wide range of possibilities in birth-giving can help us better understand our own culture of birth. We can see what is missing for women today and can work to enrich our birth culture.

This book is about rediscovering the power of women's bodies, the support that women can give each other, and the vital importance of the skilled midwife who is a specialist in physiological, rather than medical, birth.

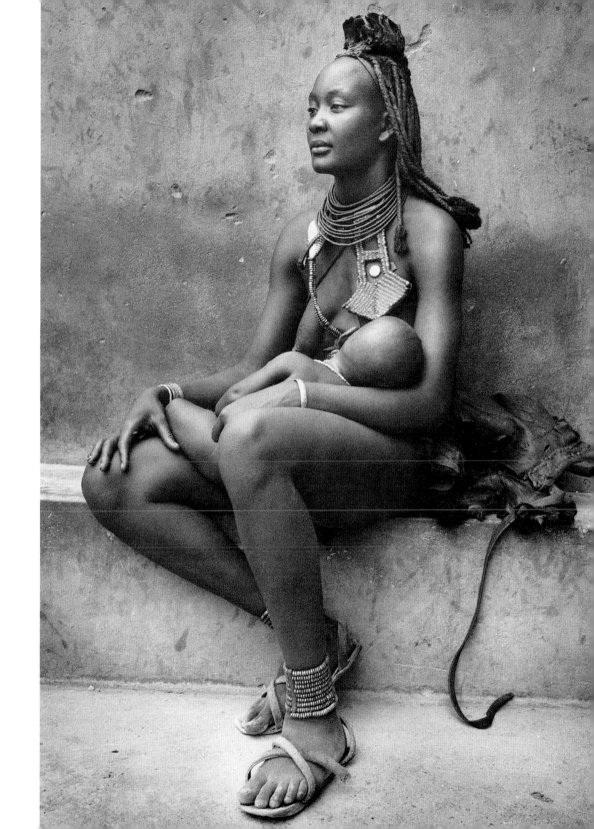

Right: A Himba woman breastfeeding her child in Opuwa, Namibia.

Chapter 1

A Small Miracle

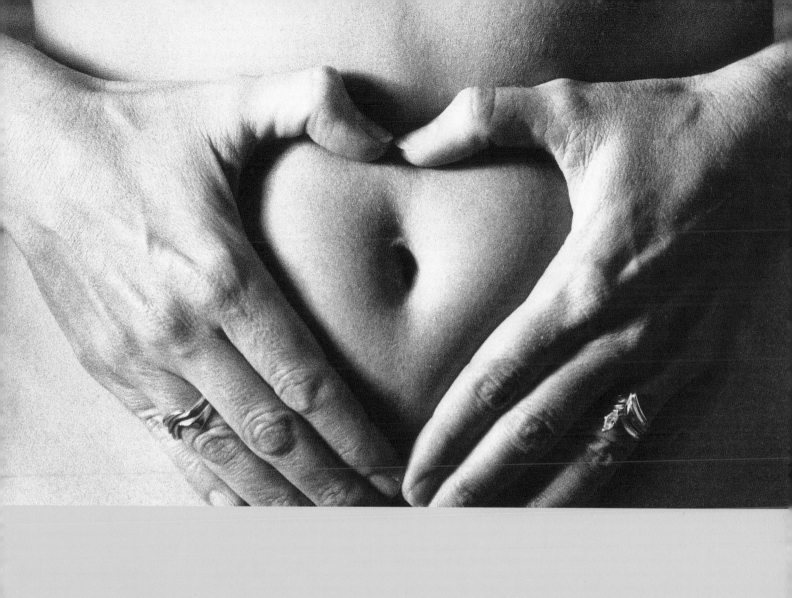

A wanted pregnancy: for any woman the meaning of what it is to be with child has its roots in their culture. A pregnancy may be proof of womanhood, a sign of a man's strength, the seal on a relationship, acceptance by a man's family, and an important stage in the interlaced network between different families. It may represent the fruit of romantic love, fulfil an aching desire to become a mother, be a symbol of hope for the future, entail the reincarnation of an ancestor, replace a child who has died, and, as throughout Africa and the Indian sub-continent, promise another hand to carry water and firewood, to weave cloth, or to shepherd the goats and till the land. Pregnancy can mean all these things, and more.

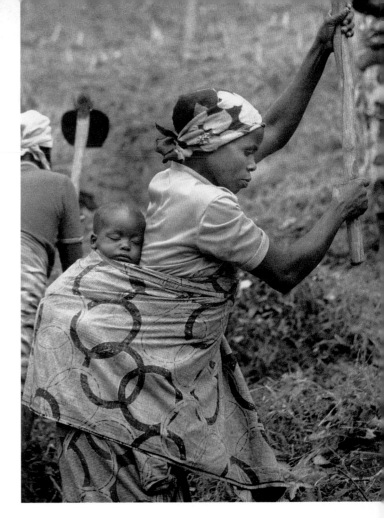

A woman may discover she is pregnant because she has been timing her menstrual periods or counting her 'moons'. Perhaps her mother observes early physical changes – her nipples have darkened and the little bumps around them on the areola are more pronounced – and tells her that she must be pregnant. She may have nausea or sickness (this occurs in some cultures, but not in others), start to dislike certain foods, or be especially tired. Maybe an ancestor appears in a vision and confirms that she is with child, or she dreams of a sea teeming with fish or a ripe melon bursting with seed, as in rural Jamaica. In some native American tribes the mother or father dreams of birds or puppies, a sign that conception has taken place. A Thai woman dreams of a baby boy or girl, and even about the baby's personality. Perhaps a doctor tells a woman she is pregnant, or some crystals in the pregnancy test she bought at the chemist tell her with their changed colour.

When women dream or fantasise about their babies they have confidence in direct communication with them, unmediated by the medical profession. They are in intimate contact with the life growing inside them and everybody else is secondary to that relationship. Once science and technology take over, that sense of living communication is affected by the various observations recorded by professionals. These can be used to reinforce the mother's awareness of her baby, but they often impose another order of reality that negates the mother's own intuitive knowledge.

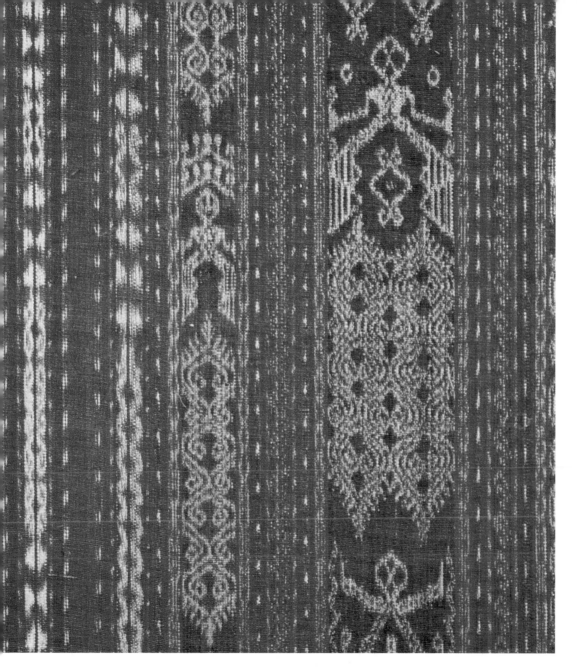

Far left: A woman working in the fields near Rumonge, Burundi.

Left: A 'birthing cloth' of warp ikat from the Philippine island of Mindanao.

In many Third World cultures human pregnancy is believed to be the force that makes the crops grow and animals bear young. There is an interconnection between human fertility and the productivity of nature. They are both part of a greater organic whole. The fertility of the land and of the animals and the spoils of hunting depend on human fertility. When women in the village are pregnant all will be well with the harvest and the food supply.

There is an element of truth in this, for when women are starving ovulation ceases and they only become fertile again when they are consuming enough calories. Menstruation fails in anorexic women, often one of the first symptoms of an eating disorder to be recognised. Even when the diet is just above the basic level there is an increase in miscarriages, preterm births and fetal abnormalities.

In some cultures pregnancy is announced as soon as it is revealed. In Fiji, for example, everyone greets the news with gladness, discusses it, exchanges advice and comments on the woman's state of health and her growing belly through the following months. It is the responsibility of the whole community to nurture the pregnancy.

Traditionally, among the Maori in New Zealand a female choir sings to the baby and the expectant mother about the progress of her pregnancy. If things are not going well or they detect signs that the baby is not developing normally they sing about this, too, in the *marae*, the great wooden temple in

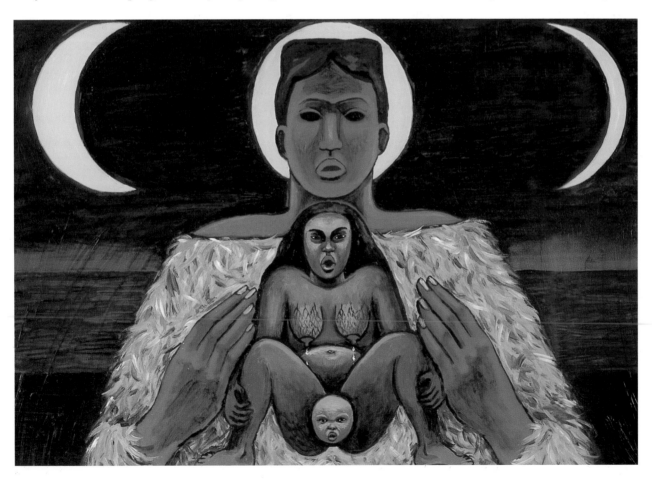

which the communal life of the people is conducted and which represents the spirit of the tribe. Each pregnancy links women together in shared pleasure or concern.

In other cultures discussion of pregnancy is avoided. The woman must disguise her changing shape and carry on with her work just as she did before. This used to be the case in rural Greece – in order to have a healthy, beautiful baby, pregnancy had to be hidden – and until very recently in the rural west of Ireland, too. An expectant mother must not 'give in', and if she lay around and was thought to be exploiting her pregnant state, she came in for a great deal of criticism from her mother-in-law and was despised by the neighbours.[1] It was a stoic ideal which stemmed from the philosophy of Irish Jansenism: a 'real woman' gets on with her work without complaint, never draws attention to herself in any way, and gives birth without fuss, unlike the 'tinker women' who moan and cry out.

Taking an unborn baby for granted, talking about it as if it were already there, collecting a layette, buying equipment for the baby, and especially bringing the cot or pram into the home, is a risky procedure which is believed to attract the attention of evil spirits, or, throughout Europe and North America, negative influences at least. Vietnamese women avoid mentioning their due date, while Hmong women (refugees from Laos and Vietnam living in the USA) are very uncomfortable about announcing the expected date of birth when case records are filled out in prenatal clinics.[2]

In the Jewish tradition women often kept a pregnancy secret, and many Ashkenazi Jews still feel happier doing so. But in the Ottoman Empire Sephardic Jews celebrated with a pregnancy rite, *Kortadura de Fashadura*, 'the cutting of the swaddling bands', when women gathered together to make the first swaddling cloth. The pregnant woman threw on to it sugared almonds to represent the sweet life that she wished for her baby.

In many cultures, an announcement of pregnancy, whether made just within the family or to a wider community, takes place only after three or four months have passed and the risk of miscarriage is reduced, or when the pregnancy is starting to become obvious.

Left: 'Breathe
help me as the next generation carves a pathway from my body.
   Breathe
in this space between worlds I link my life and yours.
   Breathe
each physical exertion pushes you toward my arms.
   Breathe
in vigour and action.'

Maori poem by Roma Potiki

Quickening

Faint fetal movements, like butterflies fluttering their wings or little fish swishing their tails, are first felt any time between sixteen and twenty weeks, although the baby has been moving without the mother being able to feel it from the twelfth week. Ultrasound has revealed that the fetus moves parts of its body in a voluntary and spontaneous way. It turns its head, waves, kicks, flexes and extends its neck, back and feet in bursts of activity. It plays with its fingers, sucks them, and plays with its mouth and umbilical cord.[3]

In all cultures, quickening is recognised as an important transition in the process of becoming a mother. In Bulgaria it is the point at which a woman would bake bread and take it as an offering to the church, letting everyone know that she was pregnant. It is as if from the moment of quickening the baby has personal identity and a life of its own, though still entirely dependent on its mother. It is an experience which only the mother can know. She is not told that it has occurred. As a direct result of her personal awareness of her baby, she is literally 'in touch' with the child.

In many religions abortion is not considered a sin unless quickening has taken place. Once a woman has 'felt life' it is a violation of the ethical code of virtually every religion. From that point on soul has entered the baby who has acquired personhood, however rudimentary that is. Since this does not happen until sixteen to twenty weeks of pregnancy, the baby is only a *possibility* until then. In most cultures, if a woman starts to bleed before there is evidence of movement, she is unlikely to mourn. It is as though the first kicks felt by the mother are a bridge between being and non-being.

Historically in Europe, women often delayed telling anyone else about a pregnancy before they felt quickening. In fact, they may not have been at all sure themselves that a baby was on the way until then. 'Quick' is old English for 'alive', as in the phrase 'the quick and the dead'. Even then, the baby was always a surprise. A woman didn't know its sex. She couldn't be sure it was perfect. She certainly didn't know what it looked like. That was part of the excitement. The birth of a baby was the birth of the unknown.

From the 17th century onwards, Englishwomen who had the education to enable them to read and write often kept journals during pregnancy and noted the first time they felt the baby kick. Quickening was a highly significant event in the pregnancy. From then on the baby inside them was 'alive'. Anne Clifford, in her diary in 1619, wrote: 'I began to think I was quick with child so I told it to my Lord (her husband), my Sister Sackville, and my Sister Compton.' In 1657 Ralph Josselin recorded in his journal

Right: Fetal movements are first felt between sixteen to twenty weeks. Later feet kick, the head bumps and sometimes there are whole body rolls.

that when Jane, his wife, felt quickening, 'the women met with her in prayer'.[4] Two centuries later Kate Amberley recorded in her diary in 1867, 'I quickened today.'

In non-technological cultures women get to know their unborn babies through awareness of their movements. It is not just how often the baby moves, but how long the movements last, their vigour and the part of the baby's body which is active – the feet kicking, the head bumping against the pelvic floor in the last weeks of pregnancy, and sometimes whole body rolls. They may notice that their babies respond to certain types of music and loud sounds, especially music with a strong beat and reverberation, such as comes from a brass band or amplified pop music, and sudden explosions as from fireworks. They know they are likely to start kicking when they lie down and try to sleep, because a baby can then move more easily, free of the curve of the mother's lumbar spine. In late pregnancy a baby's energetic activity can reassure a mother that she is bearing a healthy child, though complete body rolls and somersaults are impossible once the baby is a tight fit in the pelvis.

Visualising the Unborn

Aristotle claimed that the baby had experience inside the womb. An Indian sage of the 6th century BC, Susruta, taught that the fetus experienced its environment from the 12th week of pregnancy, and Caraka, the great medical philosopher, writing in 1000BC, and later Empedocles in Greece, in 450BC, described how the baby might be affected positively or negatively by the mother's mental state.

European medical illustrators and modellers of the unborn baby managed to render the mother's body as a transparent container for the fetus. They also devised a method by which her belly could be opened up, rather like slicing the top off a boiled egg, or – another solution – they got rid of her as a person altogether, and only showed the fetus.

The ancient Chinese taught that the baby in the uterus passed through stages in which it looked like different Buddhist ceremonial icons, weapons and charms, symbolising phases in the development of the soul to this life. Women who miscarried must have known that the unborn baby looked nothing like these objects. But the books were written by men. What they lacked in first-hand knowledge they filled in with theory.

The first carefully observed and realistic surviving illustration of a baby curled up in the uterus, encased like a kernel inside a nut, was by Leonardo da Vinci. Subsequently, da Vinci produced a drawing that showed a blood vessel running from the mother's uterus to her breasts through which blood flowed and turned into milk. It does not really exist, but conformed to the contemporary myth that the mother's blood was transformed into breastmilk.

Other illustrations omitted the shape of the uterus and depicted the baby with long limbs, like an adult in miniature, with a relatively small head and full-sized adult male genitals, jumping about in all sorts of postures, some of them very unlikely, as if inside a circular play-pen or, perhaps, on a jungle training course.

From the Middle Ages on, the mother was often rendered invisible.

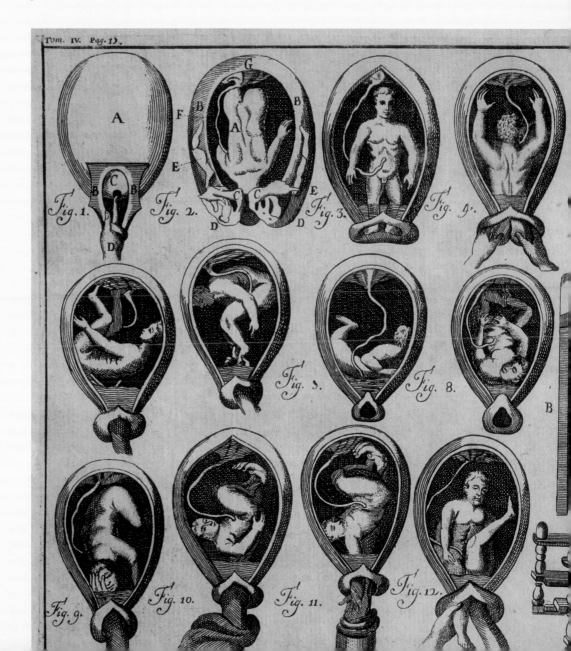

Left: 'The infant and womb' by Leonardo da Vinci.

Right: The baby was depicted with a small head and long limbs, like an adult in miniature, jumping about vigorously. From Lorenz Heister, *Institutiones chirurgicae* (1740).

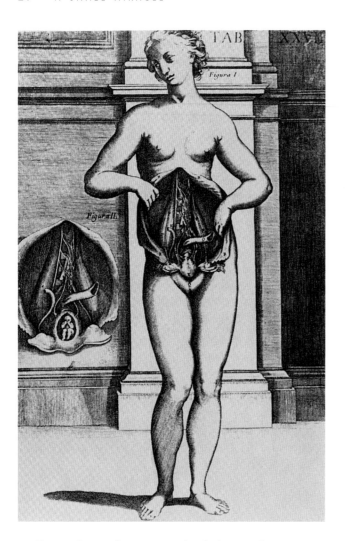

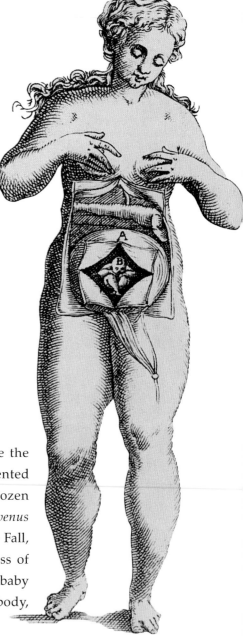

Left: The classical nude, frozen in immobility. From Petro Berrettini, *Tabula anatomicae* (1741).

Right: The *venus pudica* – a goddess displaying her ripped open pelvic cavity. From Scipione (Girolamo) Mercurio, *La comare o riccoglitrice* (1601).

From the 16th century the baby in the uterus was sometimes depicted inside the body of a woman who was usually highly romanticised. These images represented stereotypes of women as seen through men's eyes.[5] There is the classical nude, frozen in immobility, the courtesan exhibiting her charms to a man's erotic gaze, the *venus pudica* – a goddess displaying her ripped open pelvic cavity, and Eve before the Fall, holding the apple with which she will tempt Adam to take a bite and bring loss of innocence and the knowledge of evil to humanity. In Spieghel's drawing the baby appears surrounded by petals formed by the dissected tissues of the woman's body, and there is also the lily of the annunciation, a sign of redemption.

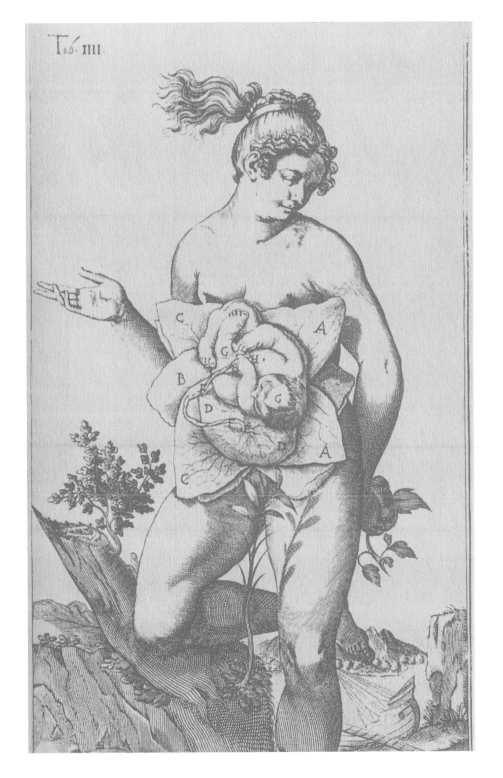

Left: From Adriaan Spieghel, *De formato foetu* (1626). The baby is surrounded by petals formed by the dissected tissues of the woman's body.

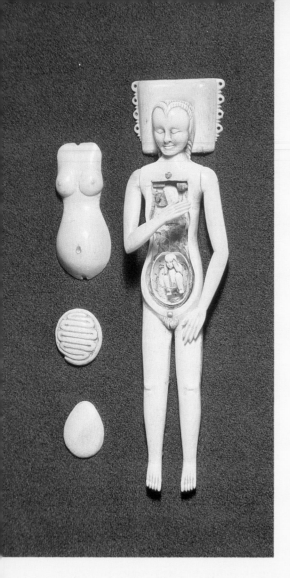

In Renaissance Italy, anatomical wax figurines of men and women were created in which nerves, muscles and all the internal organs were put on view in meticulous detail.

In the 18th-century wax anatomical collection in Bologna, women recline in sensual abandon. They are straight from the pages of the erotic romance. The woman is the seductress who now lies literally exposed, with the fetus, the fruit of her sin, revealed in her dissected body. Or she is dressed in silk finery, frills and jewels, with a prim expression on her face,

Below: *La Venerina* — the seductress lies literally exposed, with the fetus, the fruit of her sin, revealed in her dissected body.

Above: An anatomical wax model of a pregnant woman with removable parts.

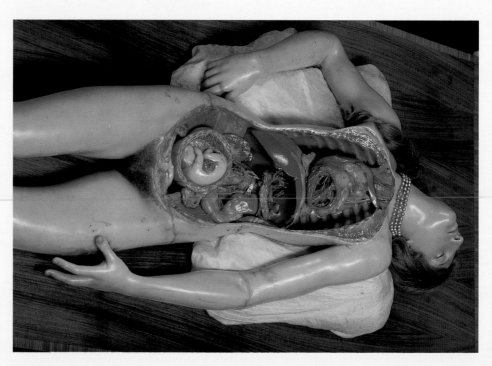

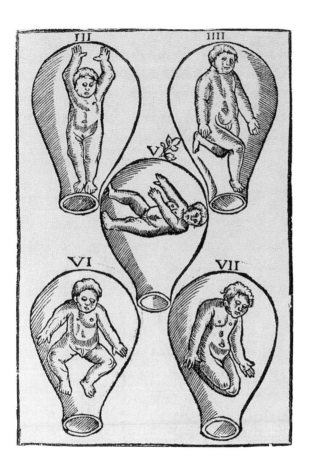

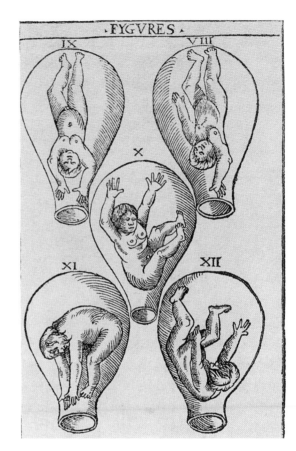

Above: From Eucharius Röesslin, *The Birth of Man-kinde*. The baby rolls, thrusts and leaps in an excised and vase-shaped uterus.

smiling coyly like a Dresden mantelpiece shepherdess with the baby curled inside her. It is as if she were carrying a handbag and was unaware of its contents. Her pelvic cavity has been ripped open, and a fetus lies inside it. It produces the sense of shock one gets from the contemporary British artist Damien Hirst, who pickled a cow cadaver in formaldehyde and displayed it in a glass cabinet. Whatever the artistic convention, the pregnant woman is depicted as entirely passive and the baby (invariably male), rolls, thrusts and leaps within what is often an excised and vase-shaped uterus. It is as if the uterus were an organ independent of all others, disconnected from a maternal heart, circulatory system and lungs – and clearly deriving no benefit from a woman's brain. Some of these illustrations give the impression that a fetus can develop into a fully-formed human being without needing to be inside a woman.

The Ultrasound Image: another way of knowing

Today, the dominant image of the unborn baby is provided by an ultrasound scan – a splodge of dots, a mottled moonscape of barely recognisable body parts, a large bulbous head and, perhaps, stick-like arms and legs, a gaping mouth and pug nose.

By penetrating the body of the woman, ultrasound enables obstetricians to find out more about what is happening inside the uterus within which the fetus is hidden from ordinary view. With ultrasound and electronic monitoring, her uterus becomes transparent and open to gaze. Obstetric intervention is initiated acting on this information.

Ultrasound scans are routinely used to date pregnancy, to record fetal growth and to diagnose abnormalities. At least one scan is mandatory, and in countries such as Germany and Greece half a dozen or more. For the woman it is an exciting moment, when she first sees her unborn baby as a pattern of dots and fuzzy blobs on the ultrasound screen. Questions have been raised about the safety of ultrasound. Might it cause nerve damage leading to hearing problems in adulthood, for instance? Could there be minute cellular changes that result in conditions that only show up many years later? The answer is 'probably not'. But it took fifty years for the danger of X-rays in pregnancy to be acknowledged.

Since the 1920s, doctors working with X-rays were warning others about their danger in pregnancy, but it was not until thirty years later, when Dr Alice Stewart revealed that radiation of the fetus led to an increased risk of cancer before the child reached the age of ten, that the routine practice of X-raying pregnant women was stopped.

Researchers have been unable to show that ultrasound is dangerous. Yet there is a different risk. It lies in the decisions that are made and actions taken as a consequence of ultrasound, rather than any inherent danger in scanning photography itself. Certainly having a scan affects the way parents 'see' their baby. It is the projection of an image that is monitored and interpreted by medicine. The focus is on the integrity of or possible damage to developing organs, and whether the fetus complies with a standard of normal growth.

There are other problems associated with ultrasound. Firstly, it may introduce unnecessary anxiety. Scans in the first half of pregnancy often diagnose the placenta as 'low lying'. Only six per cent of these turn out to be placenta previa (lying in front of the baby's head and so likely to cause a massive bleed before the baby can be born) at thirty to thirty-two weeks. But whenever a low lying placenta is diagnosed, the woman is left to worry about it, thinking that she may need a Caesarean section or have a sudden bleed resulting in the death of the baby.[6]

There are 'false positive' findings. A 'false positive' finding is the diagnosis of a condition subsequently discovered not to exist. One in 200 women who are given the news that the baby has a defect turns out to be carrying a normal baby, or one with only minor abnormalities. As a result some healthy babies are aborted because of such a false positive diagnosis.[7]

In many hospitals women are now offered a nuchal transparency test between ten and fourteen weeks – the test for Down's Syndrome that involves scanning tissues at the back of the baby's neck. Fluid collects behind the neck of a fetus if there are chromosomal abnormalities, when it is not moving enough to distribute the fluid, or there are heart problems. The nuchal transparency test is designed to detect abnormalities so that the pregnancy can be terminated. Yet out of 90 per cent of babies with a high nuchal transparency measurement (3mm) only 10 per cent have major abnormalities. If the measurement is very high (6mm), 10 per cent of these babies are normal.[8] This test is reassuring for many mothers, but introduces anxiety for other women who go on to have a healthy baby. Even after she holds her baby in her arms a woman may never be convinced that the baby is quite normal. This, and other tests like it, may prevent the birth of a Down's Syndrome child, but the risk is that a woman emotionally distances herself from her baby or constantly worries about her child's development. It can have a lasting effect on the relationship between a mother and her normal baby.

If the fetus is revealed by real time (moving) ultrasound, the doctor or radiologist often tries to involve the mother more by saying, 'Look, it's sucking its thumb!', 'It's kicking its legs!'. There is evidence that mothers like to have a scan because it slips to the back of their minds that it is designed to test for abnormalities – they see it instead as a social introduction to the baby. A scan has come to be expected as a routine and happy event in every pregnancy. Claims have been made by obstetricians and others that seeing the image of their baby on a scan enhances mother love and helps reluctant fathers to

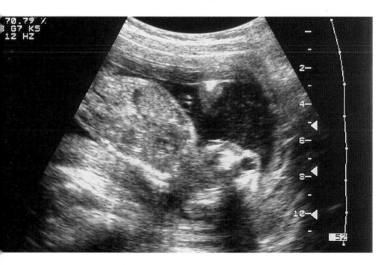

bond. Papers are published in medical journals stating that obstetricians can facilitate bonding through ultrasound, and prevent failure to bond after birth, poor family relationships, and child neglect and abuse. These obstetricians take pride in putting on a fetal performance and acting as showmen who present babies to a delighted audience. With no confidence in the spontaneous process of bonding between mothers and babies, they have taken over the task of 'promoting bonding'. They justify the use of ultrasound in pregnancy, not only on diagnostic grounds, but so that parents can bond when they see the image on the screen. It is the medicalisation of love.

Above: The ultrasound image is routinely used to date pregnancy, record fetal growth, and diagnose abnormalities.

Scientific evidence for bonding by ultrasound is dicey. Two studies of the effect of seeing a scan on women who smoked during pregnancy showed that those who had a scan were no more likely to cut down on their smoking.[9]

Having a scan is an important medical event, but it is wrong to assume that, in the absence of a scan, women find it difficult to relate to their babies until they are born. How did they get to know their unborn babies in the past? How do they still get to know them in those countries where women do not have access to ultrasound? 'Ultrasound bonding' is very different from ways in which women have always been 'in touch' with their unborn babies. It is presented and monitored by obstetricians and is under their control. The knowledge it offers is uni-dimensional, for it depends on only one of our senses – sight. And, like any photograph, holiday snap or video, it records only a fixed moment or brief period of time.

There is a world of difference between a mother's growing awareness of her baby's movements, like secret messages coming from this unborn child, and being shown an ultrasound scan. When a woman feels her baby kick she is literally in touch with her child. When she gazes at the scan, the baby is 'out there', a creature separate and removed from her body, as if alone in space. The intimacy of the relationship has gone, and other people with specialist knowledge are able to interpret the image more accurately than she can. Anyone can watch the fetal movements and these can be verified in a way that a pregnant woman's own descriptions of movements cannot. This is based on the assumption that everything the mother feels is subjective, while everything that can be produced by technology is objective, scientific and measurable. Diagnosticians may withhold information from her because they believe either that she is incapable of understanding it, or that information which indicates that there is something wrong with the baby will worry her. If she doesn't seem very interested in the picture on the screen, they may say, 'Look, baby's waving at you!'. They control the information and the way in which the unborn baby is introduced to both parents.

In law, the baby in utero is in such a close and intimate relationship with the mother that it is treated as part of her body, as much as her hands, legs or breasts. It is not yet a person 'in its own right'. Legal cases resulting from court-enforced Caesarean sections have underlined the ruling that a woman cannot be compelled to accept medical or surgical intervention for the sake of the fetus. Her body is inviolate. Yet increasingly, visualisation of the unborn child, sometimes just for the warm thrill of seeing that a baby is really

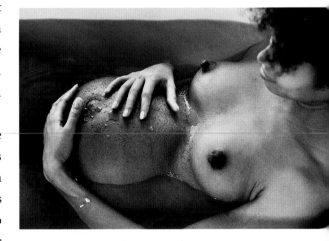

Above: When a woman feels her baby kick she is literally in touch with her child.

there in the dark cavern of the woman's body, brings the fetus to the surface, removes it from the mother's uterus and places it on film for critical inspection. Some women yearn for this. Others are uncertain. Still others want to hold the baby inside them to clasp their secret. Different women will want different things.

The latest technological development is the 3D picture of the fetus. At last the baby has a human face with a facial expression in which, for example, family characteristics can be detected. Parents can buy video copies of this to take home, and instead of a splodge of dots, a mottled moonscape of barely recognisable body parts, can observe a little creature floating in amniotic fluid like an astronaut in a space capsule. This new kind of scan enables doctors to watch the fetus as if it were a tiny actor on a TV screen, and pick up abnormalities earlier than if they were using conventional 2D ultrasound scanners, and in more detail. It means that termination can be carried out earlier, or that sometimes fetal surgery may be attempted to correct an abnormality. Then a classic Caesarean section is performed to access the fetus, which is operated on and replaced in the mother's uterus. At present some 50 per cent of all babies die when fetal surgery is performed. It is difficult to assess how many of these babies would have died shortly after birth, or survived with disabilities.

Once science and technology take over, the sense of living communication between a pregnant woman and the baby inside her is bound to be affected by the measurements, assessments and other observations that are recorded by professionals. Ultrasound has revealed a great deal about how babies behave inside the uterus. This can be used to reinforce the mother's sensitive awareness of her baby. But, in effect, ultrasound in a modern medical system often imposes another order of reality that negates the mother's own knowledge.

Ultrasound and the Longed-for Son

In many traditional patrilineal cultures, sons are wanted because they carry on the family tradition and the family name, devote their labour to the family of their birth, bring in a woman's dowry when they marry, and have the responsibility of caring for elderly parents. Daughters, on the other hand, marry 'out', and will give their work and bear their children for some other family. They are also a financial liability because puberty, marriage and birth rituals entail heavy expenditure and the family must raise a dowry that they can take with them into marriage. If a woman has daughters and no son she is seen as a reproductive failure, however many children she has. The birth of a son is greeted with celebration; the birth of a daughter with muted pleasure or dismay.

This is how it is in India, especially in the south and the north-east among land-owning communities such as the Rajputs and the Jats. When a baby girl is born the parents have to decide whether to 'keep' it. A proverb in Tamil Nadu has it that 'Bringing up a girl is like watering someone else's garden'.

Now, in urban areas of India, ultrasound in early pregnancy has made it possible to diagnose the gender of the fetus and to abort an unwanted baby. The Indian Government passed a law in 1994 making it illegal to terminate a pregnancy purely on the grounds of sex. But the law goes largely disregarded and there are rich pickings for obstetricians in sex diagnosis and subsequent abortion. The advertising has changed from: 'Pay Rs500 now [the cost of an abortion] and save Rs5,000,000 later [the cost of a dowry]', to 'Healthy boy or girl? Find out now'. Abortion clinics flourish and advertise openly, and the practice of sex selection abortion is on the increase. Because the law prohibiting this practice has been passed, doctors feel justified in putting the cost up, and many also make money from bribes.[10]

The ethical dilemma facing those who campaign against the practice is that if a pregnancy involving a female baby is not terminated, the alternative may be infanticide. The newborn baby is smothered, left exposed in the forest, or simply not fed. Parents may be under pressure to get rid of a female baby because this is yet another mouth to feed and extreme poverty puts the other children at grave risk. Women may be ordered by their husbands to have sex selection tests and are reluctant themselves to give birth to a girl since this will downgrade them in the family and make them more vulnerable to abuse. They also realise that a daughter may face a life of misery. But whatever their own wishes, they usually subordinate them to the needs of the family. The upshot is that the combination of modern technology and traditional family values results in the use of medical technology to reinforce a system of discrimination against females and their virtual murder.

Prior to the introduction of this technology a woman might guess that she was pregnant with a boy because she dreamed of a fruit or a flower, or that she was having a girl because she dreamed about a vegetable. Girls were conceived during the dark phase of the moon and boys during the bright phase. A woman carrying a daughter had blacker nipples, her abdomen bulged more, the uterus was elongated, and the baby lay on the left side. With a boy her nipples were lighter and the baby lay on the right side. The mother's psychological state was also believed to be affected by the baby's sex: she was more active with a boy and preferred mild, sweet food, whereas if it were a girl she felt lethargic and liked spicy food and pulses. But there was such uncertainty about these signs that very few abortions took place. The ready availability of ultrasound has replaced guesswork with certainty and enabled the abortion of female fetuses to be undertaken with confidence.[11]

In a north Indian village near New Delhi, where female babies have in the past often suffered fatal neglect, it has been estimated that women have between one and three abortions a year to achieve 'the ideal family'. One woman said, 'In order to get a son the mother should be ready to undergo a lot of hardship, even face death. Once she gives birth to a son, everything will be all right and all the hardship will end, but if she does not have a son, her life is better not to have been lived.' This community has responded to increasing urbanisation by reducing their family size and increasing the ratio of boys to girls, choosing to have two sons and then a daughter.[12]

Until the 19th century many tribes in India practised shifting cultivation. This was mainly women's work and men had a minor part in the rural economy. There was no dowry system. In contrast, when a woman married, her husband's family had to pay a bride price. Girls were economically valuable. Under British rule these tribes were made to turn to settled agriculture and previously communally owned land was parcelled out between male heads of families. Women had no rights in land and became entirely dependent on their husbands and sons. Now scarcity of land has increased the value of sons, and as the society becomes increasingly urbanised those who do not become farmers are sent away to be educated, since sons with high status jobs are basic to upward social mobility. There still exist tribal people for whom payment of a bride price is the norm, but this is rapidly changing and they too are shifting to a dowry system.[13]

This is an example of how the introduction of modern technology to a traditional society combines with socio-economic change to present new problems and to cause increased violence against women.

Growing a Healthy Baby

The idea that the baby *in utero* can be affected, both physically and psychologically, by what the mother sees, hears and thinks, is ancient and universal. A pregnant woman should be serene. She must avoid stress and anxiety and her wishes should be satisfied. Everyone around her has a responsibility to create a harmonious environment. Traditionally, in many Jewish communities it was believed that a pregnant woman should see only beautiful things.

In the Brahman era in India (800BC–1000AD), women followed the advice of two famous doctors, Caraka and Susruta, to avoid all anxiety, anger, tiredness, excitement, sudden noise and any emotional disturbance in case the baby was harmed by the mother's distress.

The oldest surviving medical text that includes guidance about pregnancy is the Chinese *The Fundamentals of Medicine* or *Ishin-Ho*, dating from 984AD. There are thirty volumes altogether, five of which were translated into Japanese in 1692 and published as *A Useful Reference Book for Women* or *Onna Chohoki*. It teaches that fetal development is affected by a pregnant woman's diet and by what she sees and feels. There are recommendations for each month of pregnancy.

Japanese beliefs about pregnancy are all Chinese in origin. *Taikyó* is the way in which an expectant mother should concentrate her life force to 'create a sage'. The Japanese dictionary definitions of the word *taikyó* are as follows: 'Education for unborn children. A woman should try to sit straight, to have a correct diet, to see no evil, to listen to good music and suitable counsel in order for her to provide a good influence for her unborn child'[14]; 'During her pregnancy a pregnant woman maintains her mental and emotional calmness and trains herself to behave better so that she can provide a favorable influence for her unborn child'.[15]

The word *taikyó* consists of the kangi characters for 'teaching' and 'womb'. These two characters were already combined in China, and the ancient *Daikanwa* dictionary offers the story of the Chinese empress Tai-zan who lived in the 13th century BC and who 'commenced the instruction of her child when he was still in her womb'.[16] Tai-zan had the sages of her court instruct her child as if it had already been born and could hear and understand.

In many cultures, the mother's mental state is believed to affect the baby not only psychologically, but physically. If she does not have the food she craves, the fetus may be marred. If she wants strawberries, for example, and does not get them, the baby may be born with a strawberry mark. This is the explanation for other birthmarks that seem to look like a food or an animal. If the birthmark looks like a mouse, for example, the mother must have been frightened by one. A hare lip and cleft palate indicate that she was alarmed by a hare.

Yemenite Jewish women were given whatever they wanted to eat because otherwise the baby would be born blind in one eye or have a birthmark. Egyptian peasants today say that pregnant women often long for fish, watermelons, grapes or a vegetable, and that it is important to provide these foods in case the baby is marked by the mother's craving.[17]

Dramatic climatic changes, thunderstorms and eclipses of the sun or moon are thought to affect development, too. In rural areas of Mexico it is believed that a woman may bear a baby with a hare lip if there is an eclipse of the sun. Eclipses seem to relate to a range of beliefs about shadows. In many cultures if a person's shadow is 'lost', so is their soul. In the case of the Nahuatl people of Mexico, this belief may be more to do with their myths about how the sun and moon were created and the importance of rabbits in their culture.

In Sicily, a synthesis of ancient Greek, Roman, Arabic and Spanish beliefs about birth is still strong. When a pregnant woman has what in Sicilian dialect is called *u risin*, a craving for a food, it must be offered to her as soon as possible. If this cannot be done and she touches any part of her body, a blemish will appear on the baby's skin in the same spot. To avoid this happening she must say, '*I pì signuri, incinta sugnu!*' – 'Lord, I am pregnant!' Or she draws her fingers from her armpit down over her body and flicks them away from her outer thigh to rid herself of the possibility of a birthmark. If she sees anyone with a physical disability she prays, 'God who made this person, save me from having a deformed child', and makes a similar gesture, first touching her tongue with her fingertips. During pregnancy she also avoids wearing anything black, lest the baby be born blind. In India, in the Vedic tradition too, a pregnant woman must wear only light shades, and the best colour of all is pink.

A woman's distress at seeing someone with a physical disability, a withered arm or paralysed leg, for example, might result in the baby being born with the same condition. This has remained part of folk belief in many different cultures. The remedy is to protect her from all disturbing sights and sounds. The Onitsha Ibo of Nigeria say that a pregnant woman should not be exposed to anything ugly. If she sees someone with a physical malformation or is frightened by a monkey, her baby may be born looking like this.

In the Caribbean this is the reason why pregnant women should not see a corpse or attend wakes and funerals. In Jamaica, European books of advice about pregnancy were used by slave owners to encourage vigorous breeding from the 17th century onwards. The European beliefs mingled with those of much older West African birth cultures and it is believed that the coldness of death may slip from a corpse directly into the unborn baby, that the shock felt by the expectant mother can cause miscarriage, premature delivery or the birth of a baby who is very frail.[18]

A midwifery book published in England in 1637, *The Expert Midwife*, gives counsel to pregnant women, and as well as avoiding funerals, advises: 'Let them take heed of cold and sharp wind, great heat, anger, perturbations of the mind, fears and terrors, immoderate Venus, and all intemperance of eating and drinking.' It continues 'that no peril and danger may happen to them which are with child by any manner of means, either by sudden fear, affrightments, by fire, lightning, thunder, with monstrous and hidden aspects and sights of men and beasts, by immoderate joy, sorrow and lamentation, or by intemperate excess emotion of running, leaping, riding, or by surfeit or repletion by meat and drink, or that they being taken with any disease do not use sharp and violent medicines using the counsel of unskilful physicians'.[19] That is pretty comprehensive advice, and covers a wide range of possible causes of fetal abnormality.

As late as the 19th century in England doctors advised that pregnant women should be relaxed and mentally composed to avoid the baby having a physical deformity. An article in *The Lancet* recommended a daily rest in a quiet, cool room, 'in order to keep their sensibilities calm less the baby become imprinted with harsh positions or disfigurements'.[20]

This was challenged by Joseph DeLee, the Chicago obstetrician and author of *Obstetrics for Nurses* (1904): 'Most physicians do not believe that the state of the mother's mind during pregnancy can affect the fetus. They base this disbelief on the fact, which cannot be doubted, that there exists no connection, either nervous or vascular, between the child and

Above:
A West African carving of a pregnancy doll

its mother. ' However, he went on to say: 'If a woman believes that by reading good books her child will be intellectual; that by studying good pictures and sculpture a child will be artistic; that by engaging in the science of mechanics her child will be mechanical, the belief may be encouraged, as it conduces to the welfare of both, even though there is no scientific basis for the belief.'[21]

Today many pregnant women believe that they can communicate with the baby inside them and affect the baby's character in a positive way. Japanese parenting magazines are packed with articles about how talking to the baby or playing music, massaging the uterus and touching the different parts of the baby can raise a baby's IQ level and might even produce a genius. This idea also exists in the West. There is one particular American approach to prenatal education, for example, called 'The University of the Womb'.

Maybe there has always been something in 'old wives' tales' that connects the psychological welfare of the mother with a positive pregnancy outcome. We are only beginning to discover the intricacies of interaction between the mother and the baby in utero. For example, research is accumulating on the effects of stress on the pregnant woman, and how this transfers to her baby. In some of these studies, maternal stress has been equated with going out to work. Researchers have claimed that, for some women at least, paid employment imposes stress on pregnancy, and some have drawn the conclusion that pregnant women ought to stay at home, as if a woman might not find housework and child care stressful and enjoy getting to the office or factory because it promises a break from it. Knowing about this research is likely to make a woman who has little or no choice about working feel under still more stress. As research into post-traumatic stress disorder has shown, the most threatening stress is that in which you are completely helpless and nothing you can do about it will make any difference.

Professor David Barker at Southampton University first made a link between the quality of the uterine environment and heart disease in adults, who, as babies in the uterus, suffered growth retardation.[22] Peter Nathanielsz, a Professor of Veterinary Medicine at Cornell, has demonstrated that in pregnant rats maternal stress floods the blood with a stress hormone similar to the hormone cortisol in human mothers, and that this passes to the fetus. The way the baby's system responds produces changes which are likely to cause disease in adult life.[23] If this is the case, many illnesses which are now attributed to lifestyle – cardiac diseases and diabetes, for example – may be due, at least in part, to poor conditions in the uterus.

Some dramatic responses to maternal stress have been revealed by ultrasound. When there was an earthquake in southern Italy it was observed that fetuses were jumping around and kicking as if frantic, and they continued to be hyperkinetic for up to eight hours.[24]

Yet ultrasound itself has a direct effect on the baby, too. It produces a shrill sound that we can't hear but which is like a dog whistle to the baby, who from around eighteen weeks has a keen sense of hearing. Mothers often notice that their babies move vigorously when they are being scanned by ultrasound. It seems that maternal stress increases these intense disordered movements, and that they may continue as long as the mother is in a highly anxious state. Concern about the effects of stress on the baby while it is still inside the uterus, an important element in beliefs about pregnancy in most traditional cultures, is increasingly validated by scientific research.

The perinatal psychologist David Chamberlain points out that until recently scientists believed that unborn babies were deaf and dumb and could not possibly feel pain or react violently to a stimulus because they only had 'reflexes', and that even after birth their smiles, other facial expressions and cries were not genuine communication signals and could be ignored. As a result, babies could be operated on without pain relief, provided they were injected with drugs to paralyse them so that they could not move. They could be separated from their mothers however much they cried. They could be given bottles instead of breasts. 'For a half century now, newborns have been greeted with painful injections, skin punctures, refrigerated air, dazzling lights, stinging eye medication, were slapped to get an Apgar score, straightened out for body measurements, and had their heels lanced for blood samples. While waiting in the birth canal, some babies had their scalps pierced with electrodes.'[25] Chamberlain wrote in the past tense, but these practices persist in many hospitals today.

Far from being an inanimate doll, packaged inside the muscles of the uterus and completely out of touch with what is happening in the environment, the baby learns and communicates in utero, responding to touch from the seventh week, and from thirty-two weeks its whole body is covered by tactile sense receptors. The vestibular system which allows the baby to orientate itself in space is already well developed by twelve weeks. From fourteen weeks it drinks the amniotic fluid and responds to different tastes in the fluid. The baby is aware of light, even while the eyelids are fused between ten and twenty-six weeks, and reacts to lights flashed on the mother's abdomen.

Chamberlain believes that we need to think of babies inside the uterus as sentient, rather than just a bundle of reflexes. We cling to a 19th-century view of the fetus based on the work of theorists such as Sigmund Freud and Jean Piaget, both of whom had next to no contact with newborn babies or knowledge about life before birth. All the evidence indicates that unborn babies are capable of pain or pleasure, can express themselves and are able to communicate with their mothers.

In the early 1990s, Chamberlain wrote: 'Virtually everything we believed a quarter of a century ago has been discredited and a new Encyclopedia of Knowledge has been written about the senses, perception, cognition, communication and personality of babies, both newborn and unborn'.[26]

Chapter 2

The Journey to Birth

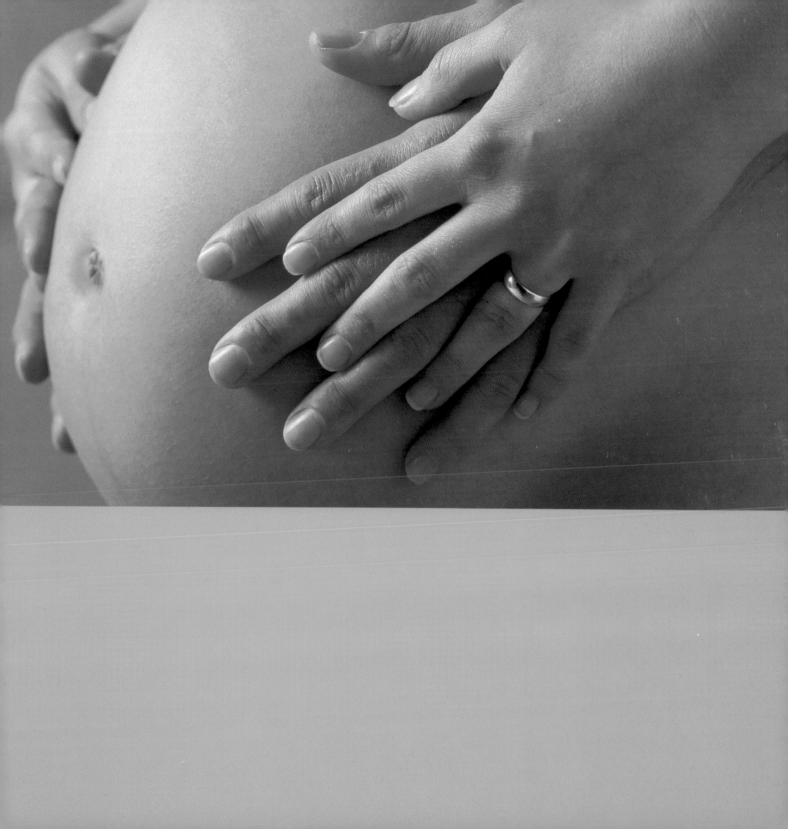

Our new knowledge about the baby in utero would come as no surprise to people in traditional cultures, where ritual acts are designed to guard the baby from being harmed by things that happen in the world outside the uterus, and to keep it safe and happy.

Pregnancy Time and Deadlines

Cultural perceptions of time in pregnancy, relating to the growth of the baby and the physical state of the mother, shape an image of pregnancy which is usually not anchored to specific states or stages, but is seen as an organic whole with its own rhythms which are independent of the calendar or of medical charts.

In some cultures, however, pregnancy ceremonies are linked to the religious calendar. In Japan, for example, the Day of the Dog in the fifth month of pregnancy, according to the Shinto religious calendar, is associated with the rite that celebrates the pregnancy and guards the baby against harm. The Dog, one of the twelve animals of the zodiac that form the ancient oriental calendar, is a messenger from the gods and chases evil spirits away. It is an auspicious time for the presentation of the expectant mother at the temple and for the donning of the *hara-obi*, the sash that protects her baby, ensures that it stays 'down' and keeps it 'warm'. She goes to the Shinto temple with her mother-in-law, and often with both prospective grandmothers, to get the *obi* from the priest and have it blessed. The women pray together at the shrine.

Only in those countries in which a medical model is dominant do women think of pregnancy as divided into trimesters. Indeed, from my own work with pregnant women it is clear that even modern women in Europe and North America are unlikely to think in these terms, though their doctors do. The pregnancy time span tends to take the form of the 'maybe' phase, then the 'announcement', followed by welcoming fetal movements and then expectation of and preparation for the birth itself. When pregnancy is medicalised, however, it is also subdivided into periods of time defined by the treatment possible and the decisions that have to be made; the first scan, the anomaly scan which reveals whether a fetus has a disability, the latest stage at which abortion is legal, clinic visits with different hospital personnel related to the progress of the pregnancy, the date from which the fetus is viable, the 'due date', the date when induction is performed for postmaturity.

Top right: In Japan, the *hara-obi* is worn by the pregnant mother to ensure the baby stays down and keeps warm.

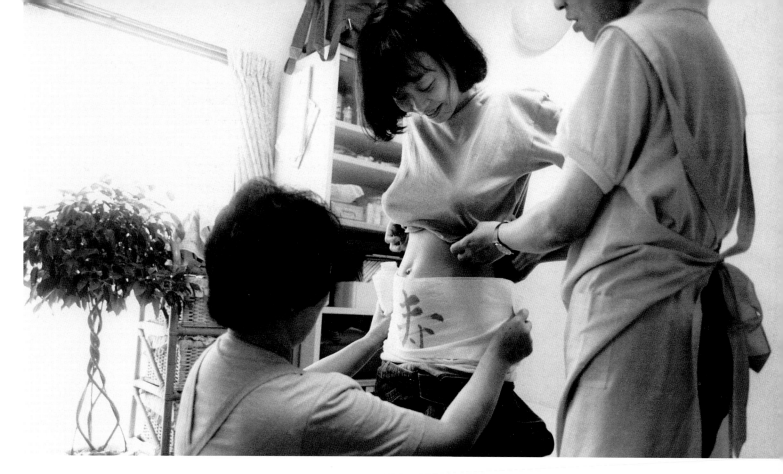

Pregnancy Rites

In Bali parents believe that they help their baby grow strong and healthy when they conduct the ceremony of *pegedong-gedoonga* ('building') around the sixth month of pregnancy. The actual time is not dependent on the calendar but is indicated when the mother starts to crave sour foods, as it is considered that the baby then has full human form. This private prayer ceremony takes place in the bathing area of the household compound. From that point on the four spirit brothers or sisters, the *kanda empot*, protect and nourish the fetus. These spirits are also born with the baby and continue to watch over the child and adult.

In India Bemata is the goddess of the life force that nurtures the unborn child just as she nurtures all plants with their roots in the earth. She lives beneath the earth and throws the baby into the woman's uterus. The *dai*, a midwife, is the 'earth mother' and works with Bemata to see that the baby is born safely. In the seventh month of pregnancy the expectant mother performs a rite in which she worships a tree and gives thanks to the spirit that lives in the tree and protects her baby by offering her sari blouse and hanging it on a branch.

Among the Navajo Hoshooji in North America the Blessing Way ceremony for 'Long-Life Empowering' is enacted during the pregnancy. It lasts nine days and involves the use of herbs, chanting and an all-night rite called 'No Sleep'. Following this, as the sun rises, the pregnant woman goes to the door and breathes deeply, visualising 'the perfect world seen by the Holy People at the dawn of the Fifth World – the world of beauty, thought, and knowledge'.[1] A Blessing Way chanter says: 'You inhale the dawn four times and give a prayer to yourself, the dawn and everything that exists. Everything is made holy again.'[2] A similar sunrise ceremony, including deep breathing and prayer, is an important pregnancy rite in South Africa among the Zulu.[3] Each morning the woman goes outside her hut and breathes deeply to empty herself of evil.

Preparing For a Safe Birth

In most cultures it is believed that a woman can also help prepare for a safe and easy birth by the way she behaves in pregnancy. In Jamaica, for example, she must avoid stepping over a donkey's tethering rope, lest the umbilical cord is drawn tightly around the baby's neck. In Sicily a pregnant woman is careful not to twist her necklace or to wear a tight scarf for the same reason. The Navajo believe that to avoid knots in the cord a pregnant woman must not sit with crossed legs.

Objects that are crossed or knotted and positions of the body that represent tightness or closure are believed to affect the way a woman's body works in labour, too, so that her cervix may not open easily. As she reaches the time when her baby is due she may be advised to undo knots in her clothing and avoid tying anything up. The Sicilian expectant mother is told to sit with her knees well apart and never to cross her legs. Everything should be open and loose. It is possible that this concentration of thinking has a strong psychosomatic effect and that it is one way of psychological preparation for birth.

Women have often sought to protect their pregnancies with amulets, charms and prayers. This remains true to this day in many cultures. Within the Christian tradition Saint Anne or the Virgin Mary are invoked. In Stuart England there were hymns and prayers specifically for pregnancy, emphasising the blessings of fruitfulness and the honour of childbearing.

In the Taormino region of Sicily, Saint Anna is the main patron of pregnancy and birth. However a male saint – San Domenico – is involved, too. On a votive card, a printed prayer to a saint, imploring his assistance and thanking him for his intervention, he is depicted as a young, smartly dressed man looking rather like the 1920s film star, Rudolph Valentino.

Russian Jewish women wear amulets. In many other religions fertility goddesses watch over women during pregnancy and birth.

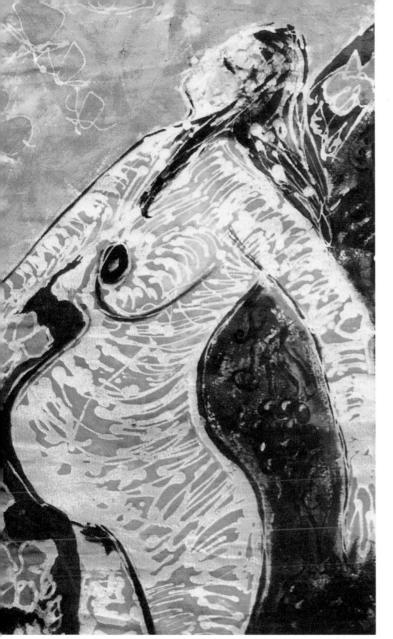

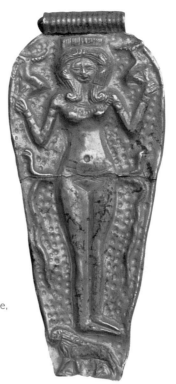

Right: A 14th-century Syrian pendant of Asarte, Goddess of Fertility.

The expectant mother may wear a pregnancy sash or belt to protect the baby. Navajo women wear a bright red sash for this purpose. In peasant Mexico, the sash, the *muñeco*, is also used by the visiting midwife to measure fundal height. The pregnancy sash often has a sacred quality. The 'girdle of Mary', worn by Englishwomen in the Middle Ages, was handed down through mothers and daughters in the family, as was the ancient Greek girdle. We have already seen that the *hara-obi* is still worn by most women in Japan today and forms part of an important ceremony for pregnant women.

In England girdles were often kept in convents and loaned to pregnant women in childbirth, too. This is how the red silk Our Lady's girdle of Bruton was used. The Jewish girdles were sometimes embroidered and later used for binding the Torah, the book of Judaic law.

The Father's Influence

In medieval times it was believed that the baby was complete in miniature within the head of the sperm, and physicians produced drawings of what they thought they saw under the microscope: the homunculus, a tiny mannikin curled up in a tear-drop capsule. It was thought that the father made the child and the mother provided the soil in which this human being could grow. Pregnancy was essentially the process of ripening; the mother was earth to the child, just as in the fields the earth offered nutrients in which the seed could sprout.

In many cultures it is believed that the father must nurture the pregnancy through his thoughts, prayers, careful behaviour and compassion; if a pregnancy fails it is felt that the father may be to blame.

When a man observes his society's rules about how he should be involved, he is making it clear that he accepts paternity and is contributing to making a healthy baby. If he ignores them, it can be taken as a statement either that he is not the biological father, that he rejects the baby as his, or that he does not care. When a man regulates his behaviour to ensure a good outcome for the pregnancy, bonds are strengthened both between the couple and between the two families concerned. It is powerful social cement.

Seen like this, rules that are otherwise incomprehensible, matters of superstition and magic, make sense, as does the male behaviour that is encapsulated collectively in the term 'couvade', invented by social anthropologists (from the French word for 'hatching'), during pregnancy, birth and afterwards. In its most dramatic form the father may enact the birth himself, making a great deal of noise and fuss about it, while the woman gives birth quietly elsewhere. More often it is he who 'lies in' and is cosseted, fed and cared for as if he has just delivered. Nineteenth-century travellers who witnessed this behaviour in the Pacific Islands, for example, were often forbidden to watch an actual birth, but were permitted to record this behaviour, and it became one of the anthropological exotica which tends to excite interest whenever childbirth is discussed.

Psychologically, the *couvade* has been explained as an acting out of male envy of the female power of giving birth. It may be more a means of deflecting the attention of evil spiritual forces away from the vulnerable mother and on to the father. In terms of social structure, it makes a public pronouncement of paternity in any society where a man's claim to fatherhood may not be clear, and where another man might well have been the biological father.

There is a tradition in Europe, North America and Japan that a father may suffer from morning sickness – even worse than his wife. It has been called the '*couvade* syndrome'. Psychiatrists have studied digestive disturbances, aches and pains, including backache and toothache, which expectant fathers complained of during pregnancy but which suddenly stopped when the baby was born. In the United States a woman said of her husband, who vomited every morning during six pregnancies: 'My man he allus does my pukin' for me.'[5] In an Oxfordshire village I learned that it was accepted, even commonplace, that a man might produce a range of ailments during his wife's pregnancy because he was 'carrying for her'.

The father must watch his step. What he does affects the unborn baby in the uterus and can make labour easy or difficult. A Navajo father must not tie up an animal. To do so may prevent the baby getting out. Many injunctions, for both expectant parents, are related to tying and untying. To give birth entails releasing all knots. If a man is careless and thoughtlessly tethers his mule or twists a rope he may have a direct effect on the birth. When labour is long and difficult a traditional midwife in peasant Greece may ask the father to undo his tie and unbutton all his clothing. Then at last the way can be made free for the baby.

Sex

Beliefs about the effects of sex in pregnancy range from cultures in which intercourse is thought to endanger the baby, to those in which it is thought to ease labour and help the baby's growth, to those in which both beliefs are held about different stages of pregnancy.

In some native American, Pacific Island and African cultures, intercourse is still forbidden throughout pregnancy. In some Muslim cultures, however, it is thought to make birth easier, and there are other African cultures in which intercourse is permitted through most of the pregnancy, though not in the final weeks. In Mexico intercourse is recommended to lubricate the birth canal and in Jamaica it is encouraged both to 'nourish' the developing baby and, as the time of labour approaches, to 'grease the passages' for birth. In Nigeria, too, semen is thought to help the baby grow and the birth to go well. The Jewish Talmud, on the other hand, recommends using a tampon during pregnancy to prevent semen reaching the cervix, while one of the earliest midwifery books published in Europe warned that strong sexual arousal could shake the baby out of the womb. These varying practices may indicate an implicit understanding that when a man has a sexually communicated disease, semen introduces infection, and also that semen can have an effect on the elasticity of cervical and vaginal tissue. Of all body fluids it has the highest concentration of prostaglandins, the hormones which, in artificial form, are used to induce labour. Like prostaglandin gel, semen can soften the cervix if it is introduced deep into the vagina. This may be a problem if a woman is at risk of preterm labour. In normal circumstances however, bathing the cervix in semen as she nears her due date may help it to ripen.

In pregnancy the cervix feels like the tip of one's nose, firm and hard. But when the woman is in a prelabour stage it feels soft and squashy, like a ripe plum. This is a sign that dilatation will start soon. When a cervix is already ripe sexual intercourse may stimulate labour contractions. Nipple stimulation also has the same effect, as the nervous system of the breast and uterus are linked.

In some cultures intercourse is encouraged in order to help the tissues of the vagina fan out. Some Nigerian tribes, for example, say that it moistens and softens the birth canal and oils the baby so that it can slip out easily. In the Philippines it is claimed to reduce birth pain, so with this in mind intercourse may take place as labour starts. When a newborn baby is thickly covered with vernix, the protective substance that looks like cream cheese that is actually produced by its own glands in utero, it is often taken as a sign that a couple have had intercourse shortly before the birth. This is approved of, laughed about, or seen as a sin, depending on the culture.

There are tribes in the lower Amazon and in New Guinea where it is believed that each man who has intercourse with a woman during her pregnancy shares biological fatherhood.

Though the husband is recognised as the primary father, every man who contributed semen is the baby's father, too. Recent studies among the Canela of Brazil and the Curripaco who live on the border of Colombia and Venezuela reveal that it is thought it takes many inseminations to make a baby, who then grows to have the qualities of the men who gave most semen. So a woman seeks out men whom she admires. The sharing of fatherhood in this way links men and families in the community and ensures that each child gains security and personal attention from a whole group of men.

Food and Drink in Pregnancy

Virtually every culture in the world is concerned with nutrition in pregnancy. From the standpoint of doctors and dieticians in northern industrialised cultures, the rules as to what should and should not be eaten in these societies may seem bizarre, but there is a logic in the recommendations even if we do not share them.

Food prohibitions in traditional cultures are often described by anthropologists as dietary 'taboos'. But by definition, when a taboo is violated it brings automatic, divine punishment. This is certainly not the case with most rules about food and drink in pregnancy. They are more concerned with foods that help the baby become strong and healthy and

> There are tribes in the lower Amazon and in New Guinea where it is believed that each man who has intercourse with a woman during her pregnancy shares biological fatherhood.

those that are thought to make the baby grow well or to stop it becoming so big that it cannot get out easily. A prohibition on eating eggs is found in many cultures worldwide. We know that egg proteins can cross from the mother's blood stream into the placenta and sensitise the fetus. When this happens the baby is born with an intolerance to or full-scale allergy to egg.

From ancient times the Japanese have had general dietary rules for pregnancy which were themselves derived from China: sweet things hinder the baby's bone formation; spicy foods unsettle the baby's soul; sour foods harm the baby's skin.[6]

Many rules about food are based on the theory of humours. A particular food can make the blood too 'hot' or 'cold'. A pregnant woman's condition must be kept in balance. The ideal pregnant state is usually seen as 'hot', so the expectant mother must avoid becoming chilled by foods that are classed as 'cold'. Hot foods are usually spicy, but some high protein foods fall into this category, too. Cold foods include most vegetables and fruits. Today, many women from Asia, the Mediterranean and central and southern American countries, believe they should avoid 'hot' foods such as chilli peppers, high salt, high fat and sweet foods, and 'cold' foods that are acidic and sour.[7] Coldness is often interpreted literally. In Sicily, for example, pregnant women avoid iced drinks because they are thought to make the baby cold.

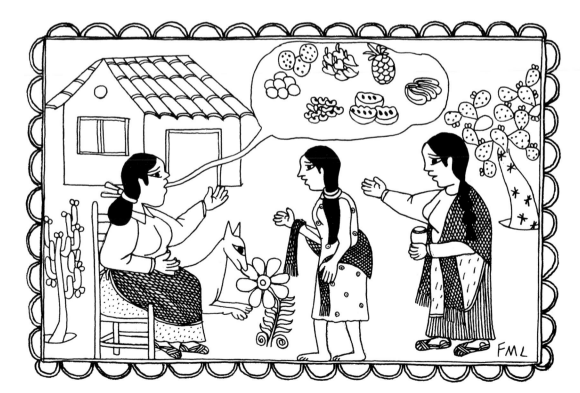

Right: Mexican *partera* recommend a nutrient-rich diet of fruit, grains and pulses to keep healthy during pregnancy.

Pregnancy is the epitome of being female, and in some cultures in Africa and Oceania, foods that are listed in the category of 'male' are also forbidden in case they cause miscarriage or fetal deformity.

Food prohibitions are sometimes linked with sympathetic magic. This is based on the idea that things that look alike are somehow causally connected. Traditionally, pregnant Japanese women are not supposed to eat crab lest it cause a transverse lie. Perhaps this has something to do with the sideways movement of a crab.[8] Ginger root is also forbidden because the baby may have extra digits sticking out like the fingers of the root. In Fiji women should not eat crab or lobster as they may cause skin eruptions, growths and tumours like the strange shapes of a crustacean.

The diets of pregnant women in other cultures are often criticised by Western doctors and nutritionists on the grounds that they are short of protein and other essential nutrients. Indian women, for example, base their diet on Ayurvedic teachings. Because pregnancy is a 'hot' condition they cut down on 'hot' foods such as meat, fish, eggs and pulses and eat mainly 'cold' foods such as vegetables and fruit. In Guatemala, women avoid very 'cold' foods such as beans, pork, avocados, some green vegetables, sodas and sometimes eggs. They also avoid very hot substances such as chilli pepper.[9]

Pregnant Vietnamese women in the United States, the Hmong, do not drink milk because it makes the blood 'cold'. This makes American health care providers anxious because milk is often considered essential in pregnancy. In fact, lactose intolerance is common among people from the Far East.

In all cultures dietary rules tend to be treated fairly lightly by individual women, who are likely to work out what suits them best. They can tell you what they 'should' eat, but what they actually eat may be quite different. Guatemalan midwives say that most pregnant women can eat everything, and it is only if they are ill that they have to avoid 'cold' foods.[10] In a detailed study of pregnancy nutrition in Malaysia, published in the 1980s, Carol Laderman reveals that poverty has a greater impact on health than any dietary rules. If a woman is well off, she is well nourished. If she is poor, she may starve.[11]

Rules about food in pregnancy are often very restrictive in contemporary northern industrial culture, too. In the 19th century American women were advised to go on a severely restricted diet in the last weeks of pregnancy so that the baby would have soft bones and be born more easily. It was believed that wheat made bone, so this was banned. Women dieted on rice, potatoes, oranges and apples, in the hope that their babies would be born with gristle instead of bone.

During the 1970s women in North America and Britain were told that eating blighted or bruised potatoes could cause major birth defects, so they omitted potatoes from their diets, just in case. The news about methyl mercury poisoning caused by eating fish and pigs fed on mercury-contaminated grain made pregnant women afraid to eat fish or pork. Fruit and vegetables might have been sprayed with pesticides. Even water was implicated in causing congenital abnormalities. Childbirth books today warn against eating rare meat, liver, red meat, soft boiled eggs, soft cheeses, peanuts and processed foods of all kinds, and drinking alcohol and even coffee and carbonated drinks. For women made anxious by these warnings, pregnancy is like walking through a minefield.

Other people have strong views about food and drink, too, and impose these on the pregnant woman. In the USA every establishment that sells alcohol is required by law to post a sign warning of the dangers of alcohol in pregnancy, and every can of beer has the warning: 'According to the Surgeon General, women should not drink alcoholic beverages during pregnancy because of the risk of birth defects.' This has come about because fetal alcohol syndrome, when the baby is damaged physically and mentally by the mother's consumption of alcohol, is a very real problem in the USA. Some birth educators tell women that those who do not give up alcohol completely during pregnancy have a serious problem.

In some communities, immediate inpatient treatment is provided for any pregnant woman who drinks any alcohol at all.[12] Expectant mothers have had alcoholic drinks snatched from their hands and replaced with juice, though there is no scientific evidence that a small glass of wine a day has any damaging effect on the fetus.

Good Things to Eat

In every culture much of the advice about food in pregnancy is positive. A woman should have a generous diet and 'eat for two', but in the last two months she should eat mainly vegetables and fruit and avoid anything that would make the baby so big that labour is difficult. Fruit and vegetables may also be advised for other reasons. In Japan it is believed that a diet high in fruit and vegetables helps the baby's skin to be clear and beautiful.

Women in Fiji are advised to eat plenty of vegetables and fish and to drink a mixture of taro and boiled cassava. Instead of ordinary tea they drink an infusion of lemon leaves. Hibiscus is also an important ingredient of potions taken in pregnancy.

At the end of pregnancy, special foods are often recommended that are thought to soften the tissues of the vagina and perineum so that the baby slips out. In the eighth month Fijian women eat the gelatinous leaves of a vegetable recommended for easy births. In Jamaica okra is recommended for the same purpose, since its gelatinous interior is believed to grease the passages to help the baby emerge.

Other foods are advised to tone the uterus, to make the woman strong, or simply, in practical ways that we can all understand, to prevent indigestion, enrich the blood or encourage lactation. Bush teas are recommended for these purposes throughout the Caribbean, Africa and Mediterranean countries. In Egypt pregnant women are told that heartburn is caused by spicy foods and are advised not to eat them. In practice they still do, since spices are a basic element in the Egyptian diet.

In Europe, since mediaeval times, herbal medications and teas have been recommended for pregnant women. Sage was known as 'the holy herb', because 'women with child if they be like to come before their time, and are troubled with abortments, do eat thereof to their great good; for it closeth the matrix, and maketh them fruitful, it retaineth the child, and giveth it life'.[13] Jane Sharpe, the first English midwife to write about pregnancy and childbirth, had great faith in sage. The renowned herbalist Nicholas Culpeper also advised women to drink sage tea to strengthen the uterus and recommended syrups of tansy and sage and boiled mallow and hollyhock.[14]

While American doctors in the 1940s routinely starved their pregnant patients, handing them low protein diet sheets in the belief that this would keep the baby small and avoid complications in pregnancy and birth, today many doctors encourage very heavy protein consumption. They claim that this is the way to prevent pre-eclampsia, though evidence for this is unreliable and diets supplemented with protein appear to be associated with higher rather than lower rates of pre-eclampsia.

In the 1960s and 1970s there was a vogue for prescribing vitamin and mineral supplements in pregnancy, and many women bought these over the counter, too. In the case of Vitamin A this was certainly not a good idea, for either in the form of tablets or fish oil drops, high concentrations can cause birth defects. For the same reason women should avoid regularly eating liver and its products, such as liver paté and liver sausage, because Vitamin A is stored in an animal's liver. But at that time, liver was promoted as an ideal food for an expectant mother.

Iron is often prescribed to build up haemoglobin in the blood. But there is a problem here, too, because iron capsules can cause gastro-intestinal irritation and nausea, diarrhoea or constipation. Women may be reluctant to take iron supplements because of the side-effects.

The great success story is folic acid, which is used for the prevention of neural tube defects in the baby (abnormalities of the spinal cord and brain). In its natural form it comes in dark green leafy vegetables, whole grains, yeast, liver and nuts. Because it is a vitamin of the B complex, together with vitamin B12, it is linked to the process of cell division, which is taking place rapidly in the developing fetus, especially at the very beginning of pregnancy. Unfortunately, women most likely to take folic acid supplements before and immediately after conception – those who are able to plan their pregnancies – are the ones least likely to need them.[15] For this reason, and because 40 per cent of pregnancies in the USA are unplanned, the only way to make sure that all pregnant women have sufficient folic acid may be to fortify a staple food, such as flour, with folates. This has already been done in the United States, but the folates are at a very low level.[16]

There remain many uncertainties about correct nutrition in pregnancy, however, and it may be that what is right for one woman is not so good for another.

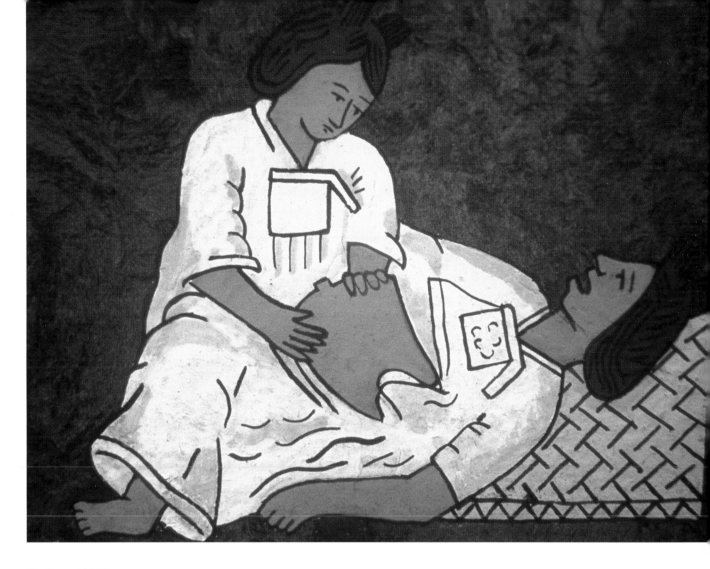

Above: A *ticitl*, an Aztec midwife, massaging a pregnant woman.

Antenatal Care

A frequent element of antenatal care in many cultures is massage. An older woman in the family, the mother or mother-in-law, for example, or the village midwife, regularly massages the woman's back, abdomen, arms and legs, using whatever vegetable oil is available locally. In Fiji and Indonesia it is coconut oil. In Mediterranean countries it is olive oil. Home visits by the midwife often include abdominal palpation at the same time as massage, while the two women talk together about how the expectant mother is feeling and how the pregnancy is progressing. At the end of pregnancy this massage may include manual rotation of a breech to vertex,

The modern medical system brought care out of the bedroom and into the clinic. Care was no longer part of the intimate relationship between a woman and her midwife, but a series of repeated investigations administered by the medical system that often took place in public.

and from a posterior to an anterior presentation. In Hawaii a 65-year-old woman described to me how her maternal grandfather massaged and turned her baby from posterior to anterior before she started labour and she had 'no trouble'.

Among Mayans in Guatemala the midwife is formally requested to visit the pregnant woman with a gift of food and money to buy candles and incense for St Anne and other saints. She visits every twenty or thirty days, and each week in the last month or so. In an easy synthesis of Christianity and preChristian beliefs she starts with a prayer to God, the spirits of orphans, widows, doctors and midwives, gives thanks to El Mundo, the spirit of the Earth and Air, the spirit of the Wind and Santa Ana, San Augustin and Santa Christina, says an Our Father and crosses herself.[17] Then she palpates the abdomen to check the position of the baby and gives a massage. She moves her hands in opposite directions across the abdomen and along the sides and may massage the woman's calves and thighs to prevent cramps and leg pains. She measures fundal height and may manipulate the baby into the best position for birth. Midwives in South American cultures listen to the heartbeat directly with an ear against the abdomen. The expectant mother may bathe her perineum (the area around her vagina and anus) in an infusion of avocado leaves and salt to make the tissues strong, soft and flexible. In many cultures she also massages her perineum. In Jamaica the oil of the wild castor oil plant and the juicy pulp of *toona* leaves are used. In Victorian England women massaged their perineums with pork fat and doctors doing vaginal examinations smeared their fingers with lard before inserting them. On hearing that I was pregnant with my first child in the 1950s, an aunt who had a baby thirty years earlier said, 'You should massage your perineum with olive oil. That's what we did.'

The modern medical system brought care out of the bedroom and into the clinic. Care was no longer part of the intimate relationship between a woman and her midwife, but a series of repeated investigations administered by the medical system conducted by a variety of professionals, and these often took place in public.

Antenatal care developed piecemeal, without much evidence that any of its interventions actually worked. It was assumed that if doctors saw women regularly during pregnancy and recorded weight increase, for example, this must lead to safer pregnancy and birth. Pregnancy could be controlled by instructing the pregnant mother to eat less or more. Great emphasis was put on regular weighing, and still is, by those doctors who believe that weight should be kept within strict limits, though there is no medical evidence to support this practice.

Formal antenatal care was first offered in St Mary's Hospital, Manchester, in 1909, and shortly after this at Queen Charlotte's, the specialist maternity hospital in London. The first regular antenatal clinic available to all women attending the hospital, not just those considered to be in most need, was started in 1915 at the Simpson Maternity Hospital in Edinburgh, though only a small proportion of patients attended it.

Urine was tested for protein, blood pressure checked to diagnose pre-eclampsia, and there were urine tests for sugar, too, in the hope of defeating pregnancy diabetes. This has been described as 'a diagnosis looking for a disease', since the presence of sugar may only indicate that the baby is going to be large, and in a normal-sized pelvis this is usually no problem. To date no way has been found of preventing pre-eclampsia, and still the only treatment is delivery of the baby by induction of labour or Caesarean section.

A great breakthrough in antenatal care was made by a maverick English paediatrician, Neville Butler, in the mid 1950s. He was the first to suggest that smoking might be dangerous after happening on an article in the *Readers' Digest* about a nursing nun in California who believed that babies weighed less when their mothers smoked in pregnancy. Later it was discovered that not only were babies, on average, lighter than those of mothers that did not smoke, but that there was an increased risk of preterm birth, damage to the placenta and fetal malformation. The problem still remained, however, of getting women to stop smoking. Women most likely to have a poor diet and to suffer from ill health – the most socially disadvantaged – were also those most likely to smoke.

Diagnosis of congenital abnormalities in the form of tests for Down's Syndrome and spina bifida was another great advance. But the only treatment is no treatment at all. The only option available is to abort the baby as soon as possible after the diagnosis is made. These screening tests pick up approximately two out of three babies with Down's Syndrome and four out of five babies with an

Right: Antenatal clinic attendance is mandatory for all pregnant women. Those who do not go regularly are classed as 'defaulters'. But we do not know if this kind of surveillance is effective, or whether for some women it may do more harm than good.

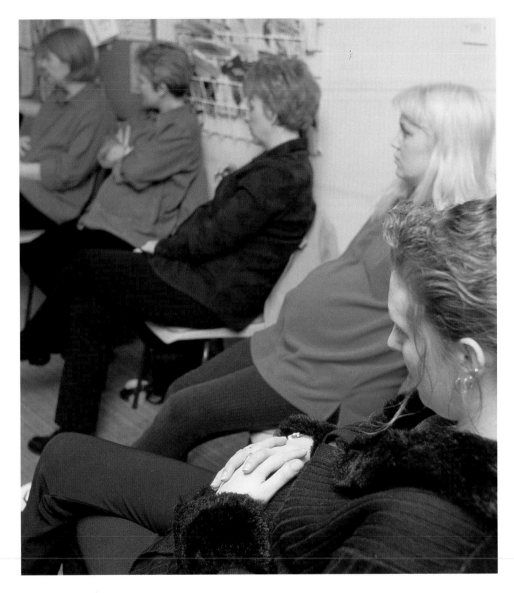

open neural tube defect, however there is always the chance that a healthy baby will be aborted.

Attendance at the antenatal clinic is now established routine for every pregnant woman. Health services invest vast amounts in the system and struggle to improve the quality of care. But they cannot claim to have achieved much success. Antenatal care has been a noble experiment which has never been properly audited. The major problems of pregnancy are ultimately a matter for public health and economic change.

The Strong, Supple Body: a pregnancy ideal

A woman's body should be powerful and lithe for birth. This belief is held in many cultures. To give birth with ease a woman should remain physically active during pregnancy, especially in the last weeks. If an expectant mother lies around it is thought her labour will be more difficult. Mexican Navajo women are advised to walk a lot to help the circulation and to keep the baby small enough to pass through the pelvis without difficulty. Women in Fiji told me that pregnant women must be careful not to sit around for a long time and should walk instead.

In Japan traditional philosophy regarding the value of hard work during pregnancy has been revived and given a new twist by an obstetrician, Dr Yoshimura, who told me that 'Pregnant women have usually finished their housework by about 8.30 am and then lie around watching TV until night time. The men don't come home until 7 or 8 pm, so women have nothing to do.'[18] He sees this as a surrender to American values introduced after the last world war: 'I seek a return to traditional ways of living. The great evil is industrialisation. Industrialisation is the cancer of mankind. We have no antibodies to it.'

Pregnant women go to his house in the early morning to do his housework, unaided by electricity or labour-saving equipment. They wash the floors, sweep and cook over an open wood fire set in a pit in the ground, do gardening and chop and saw great trunks of wood. I saw women in the final weeks of pregnancy drawing water from the well and sawing, chopping and stacking enormous quantities of wood in Dr Yoshimura's grounds.

I was invited to a meal at Dr Yoshimura's ancient house. We knelt round the open fire over which a heavy iron cooking pot was suspended in which fish and cabbage leaves were boiling. Swathed in clouds of smoke, the pregnant women attending alternately stoked the fire, producing thicker billowing smoke that made my eyes water and choked my throat, and, in response to a wave of the guru's hand, threw more fish and cabbage into the bubbling water and passed round small bowls of saki (rice wine).

Today in the West there is great concern about air pollution and its relation to asthma and respiratory diseases and cancer. It struck me forcibly that when household life is conducted in one room with a wood fire with no chimney, everyone has to breathe highly polluted air, babies and pregnant women included. This kind of ancient environmental pollution is easily forgotten but continues today over much of the world, and together with the ever-present risk of fire, is another major health risk for women and children.

When I asked Dr Yoshimura how he got women to engage in this heavy labour and endure such onerous conditions, he answered, 'I have charismatic appeal and they hear my words as from a religious master.' I was left unconvinced by his recreation of the ancient Japanese birth culture.

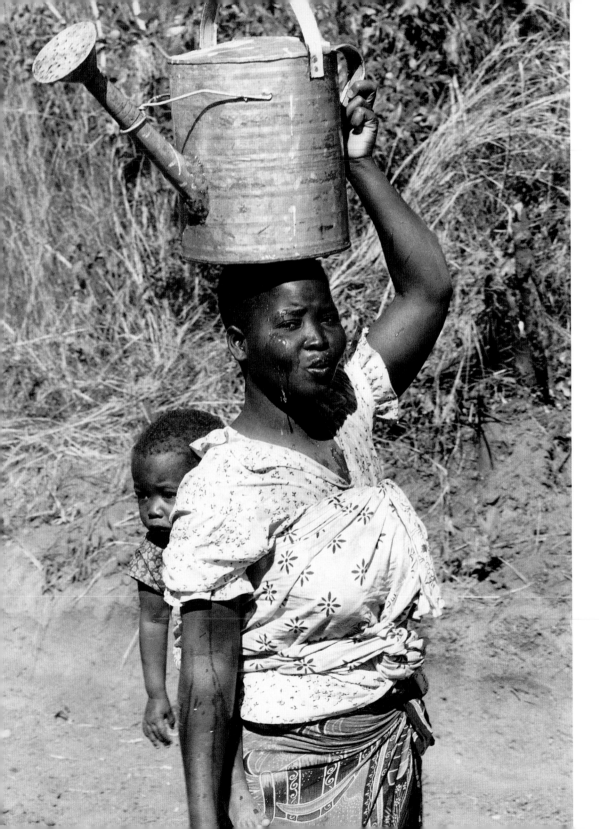

Left: Women's work all over the world includes activities that have to be performed in pregnancy as usual. If this woman did not carry water for a long distance the family would have none.

It is true that before Japan was industrialised, pregnant women in all but the wealthiest families had to face hard physical labour of this kind, as they still do in most countries. On the other hand, after a birth in traditional societies, respite from physical labour is linked with rites of postpartum segregation and nurturing by other women, and a new mother is assured a break from work and some kind of sanctuary for a short time after giving birth. Rather than wanting to 'get back to normal' as soon as possible after birth, now the norm in industrialised cultures, an Asian woman who has just had a baby expects to be cared for and to rest while others do the work. Where women come from cultures in which they anticipate a postpartum time of rest, this conflicts with the attitude of nurses who want to get the new mother on her feet, caring for the baby herself and taking responsibility in the early days following birth.

The nature of women's work all over the world – scrubbing laundry on stones in the river, drawing water from the well, picking cotton or tea, breaking up stones to construct a road – is such that it includes activities that have to be performed in pregnancy as usual. This means that most women do not have any choice as to whether they get enough exercise. In most countries throughout history, only socially privileged women have been able to rely on other women to do the work for them. The cult of antenatal exercises developed because women who were comfortably off often became physically inactive. Their muscles were untoned, circulation sluggish and bodies stiff because they no longer had to scrub floors and till the land, and because, in the 20th century, they acquired labour-saving machines that required less effort and could do at least some household tasks for them.

It is acknowledged worldwide, however, that strenuous physical work and heavy lifting is harmful in early pregnancy. Women try to avoid carrying heavy loads in the first three months, but it is often impossible in societies which are dependent on women's physical labour and where they must lift and carry fuel, water, pots and crops, and transport them for long distances. This takes a toll on their health, may cause backache and uterine prolapse and leads to miscarriage or problem births.

Throughout the Third World, women squat and kneel in positions in which the pelvis is at its widest, and in their work make movements in which the pelvis rocks, tilts and rotates in a smooth and steady rhythm. These movements, which are the basis of exercises practised in pregnancy classes in northern industrialised cultures, are elements in the daily work of rural women in South America, the Pacific Islands, Africa and the Indian sub-continent, and in the dances which universally are part of women's culture. The same movements are used when a woman is in labour, and she is encouraged by women who are helping her who rock and circle their own pelvises in the same rhythm. Bedouin Arab girls are taught these movements formally after they have had their first period, both for sex and for childbirth. What we know as belly-dancing is essentially a fertility dance in which women celebrate the power to give life.

Historically in Europe there seem to have been no specific exercises with which to prepare for birth, though what is now known as folk dance was a regular form of celebration in every rural community. After a hard week's work in the fields and the dairy, women, as well as men, gathered to dance and sing. There was advice about movement in Soranius's *Instructions for Midwives*, which was translated from Latin into German in 1513, and into English in 1540, where it was published as *The Birth of Mankind*. In this book a pregnant woman was counselled 'to exercise the body in doing something, stirring, moving, going or standing, more than otherwise she was wont to do'.[19]

In the 1920s an English doctor working in India, Kathleen Vaughan, observed that Indian women squatted, feet wide apart, in what for them was an easy and spontaneous posture, and considered that this was the reason why births she observed there seemed to be easier than for English women. A physiotherapist, Minnie Randell, publicised Dr Vaughan's ideas and the first books intended to prepare women for childbirth published in the 1930s and 1940s invariably included the suggestion that sitting on chairs was responsible for many of the birth difficulties encountered in Western countries. Expectant mothers were advised to polish shoes, darn their husband's socks, and put on nail varnish while squatting on the floor, and to use a chamber pot instead of the lavatory. Margaret Brady, whose book of advice was published in 1944, said that a woman 'should not even sit on the chamber pot, but just squat over it, supporting herself, if necessary, with her hands on something firm'. She added helpfully, 'This exercise would be hard on silk stockings, and is in fact easiest if no stockings are worn.'[20] Grantly Dick-Read, in his famous book *Childbirth Without Fear*, incorporated squatting and thigh-stretching exercises into the physical preparation for birth. He advised women to 'sit Indian-style often during the day for quiet work, reading, sewing or watching television, ankles crossed'.[21] These ideas about pelvic mobility and stretching of the inner thighs were incorporated into birth preparation classes throughout Europe and North America and formed an important part of Russian psychoprophylaxis, a vigorous system of psycho-physical training which claimed to ensure 'birth without pain'.

Expectant mothers were advised to polish shoes, darn their husband's socks, and put on nail varnish while squatting on the floor . . .

The Pregnant Body: display or concealment

In many traditional cultures women are proud to show that they are pregnant. There is no question of disguising it. In rural Jamaica I learned that when the local midwife greeted a teenager with the comment, 'You be getting fat!', it was a welcome allusion to the fact that, though she was not pregnant, she looked ready for pregnancy.

In other cultures pregnancy is hidden under tent-like clothes, perhaps as a matter of convenience, for it is easier to move and to avoid being over-heated in a loose gown. (Pregnancy has a thermal effect and women feel as if they are carrying around their own personal central heating.)

In Europe in the 19th century, the Empire line was well adapted to pregnancy and became the mode in fashionable circles. The first maternity dresses designed to draw the eye from the bump by a strategically placed elaborate collar or ribbon were made for the upper classes. These gowns were intended to disguise the pregnancy behind plackets, pleats and frills. Advertisements for dresses for the elegant expectant mother appeared in women's magazines.

Right: Maternity dresses of the 19th century were designed to disguise the pregnancy behind plackets, pleats and frills.

In 1904 an American dressmaker designed a pregnancy 'teagown' for elegant entertaining at home. It had accordion pleats all the way down from bust to ankle. This was the beginning of the Lane Bryant maternity wear store that opened its doors in 1910, advertising clothes that could also be worn out-of-doors so that women could 'go out into the health-giving air and sunshine right up to the day of confinement'.[22]

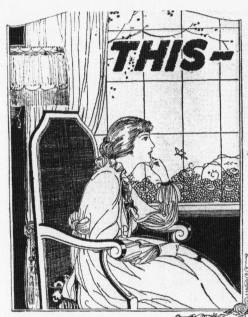
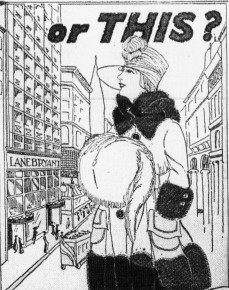

Sunshine or Shadow?
Which Do You Choose?

Here are two pictures. They are as nearly opposite as two pictures could possibly be.

One of them shows your life the next few months as it **may** be. The other as it **ought to** be. Which, dear mother, will you choose?

Will you be the "shut-in" mother? Hiding in darkness and gloom? Thinking only of things that depress?

Or will you be the carefree one? Out in the brightness and sunshine? Out where gloomy thoughts are banished? Out where friends and happiness make every day a day of joy?

You can put yourself in whichever picture you choose. And Oh, how much the choosing means to you! To choose right means a lifetime of health and happiness. To choose wrong may mean a lifetime of regret.

So choose, dear mother, with care. Choose sunshine, not shadow. Choose happiness, not gloom. Choose health, not misery.

Lane Bryant Will Help You

The choice is not easy, we know. Embarrassment tempts you to seek the shadows. False modesty urges you to hide. Pride forces you to unhealthful dress.

But pay no attention to these tempters. Cling to the other, the better way. Do as your doctor will tell you. Continue every normal activity. Lane Bryant has made it easy for you to do so.

We picture in this book a complete line of Lane Bryant Maternity garments. In these you can face the world without embarrassment. You can continue your social activities. You can go out into the health-giving air and sunshine right up to the day of confinement. You can be as proud of your appearance as you ever were in your life.

So study these garments, today. Study their beauty, their style, their marvelous figure-concealing lines, their health-promoting construction.

And then, for your own sake—for your baby's sake—take the first step on the road to health and happiness. Order now, TO-DAY, the garments that you need to drive the shadows

Left: An advertisement for the Lane Bryant maternity wear store, promoting clothes that can be worn out-of-doors.

Above right: In 1991, Demi Moore displayed her pregnant body on the front cover of *Vanity Fair* magazine, an example that was soon followed by other female celebrities.

Far right: The pregnant Spice Girls, Posh Spice and Scary Spice, meet the Prince of Wales.

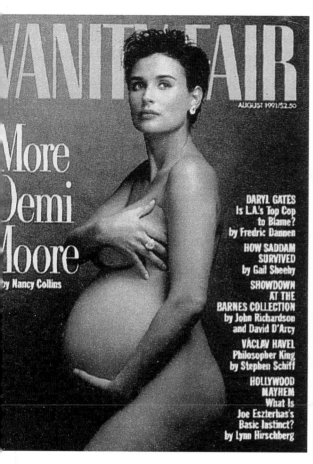

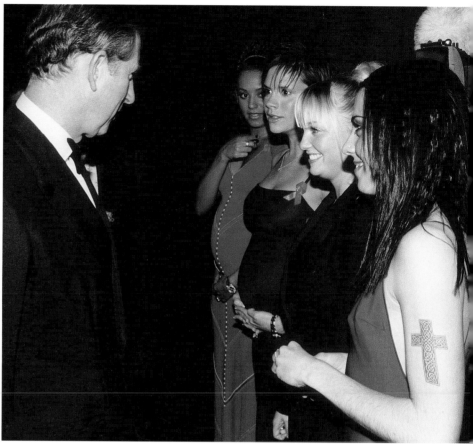

Yet many women were reluctant to submit themselves to public gaze in advanced pregnancy. In 1929, my mother, in the last months of her pregnancy, only ventured out after dark wearing a capacious greatcoat. To get exercise she and my father went for a regular evening walk. Only in the dark was she comfortable leaving the house.

It took another sixty years for attitudes to the open revelation of pregnancy to change. In the meantime maternity clothes were designed to conceal and distract, often in little-girl pinks and blues, flower-sprigged, with big bows at the neck. Women often tried to adapt their everyday clothes, but had to give up when waistbands on jeans gaped open and zips no longer worked. Then, at the beginning of the 1990s, the pregnant body was displayed in all its naked glory by Demi Moore, and her example was followed by other female celebrities. A new image of motherhood was promoted, the sassy woman in charge of her life who challenged men, even princes, with the physical revelation of pregnancy.

Women's magazines started to feature pregnancy styles with tightly fitting bodices and drop-waisted miniskirts that displayed the bump. A new image of glamorous pregnancy was promoted. Women journalists decried the old sentimental images of maternity and hailed the new icons. 'These days, of course, the ideal image of expectant motherhood is no longer the slightly narcotised blonde, deadheading roses in an English country garden . . . it's a business chick in an elasticated powersuit.'[23] Revealing party clothes of gauze and chiffon were also part of the new image, for 'being able to party when pregnant is as essential to me and my fellow society girls as antenatal classes and Tiffany teething rings'.[24]

Some of these women did not just want stylish maternity clothes. They wanted birth without pain, too. To achieve this they decided to buy a Caesarean section with the smallest, neatest bikini scar they could get, rather than have the blood, sweat and effort of vaginal birth. The question was whether the same stars who displayed their pregnant bodies with such panache would breastfeed openly. Would we see a baby suckling at a Spice Girl's breast? We did not.

Birth and the Media

When birth is reported in the media, above all on television, it is invariably an emergency. A study of the ways in which childbirth is treated in TV soap operas and other programmes on British TV reveals that labour usually starts with the waters suddenly breaking, and this is followed immediately by contractions. After the very first pain there is a rush to get to hospital, but 26 per cent of women never make it before the birth. Babies are usually delivered by doctors, not midwives, and 70 per cent of doctors are togged up in theatre gown and surgical cap, while a third wears a mask as well. 'Childbirth on television is fast, dramatic and unpredictable. In a typical fictional programme labour is heralded by the waters breaking, the mother then clutches her abdomen as powerful contractions start. There is often a chaotic rush to hospital – will she get there on time? Will her partner get there?'[25] Another writer about birth on the box comments that 'TV heroines only ever give birth in lifts, taxis, besides remote lakes or in planes, three miles up above the Earth'.[26] Home births are either historical, or if they take place in the present are unplanned and likely to result in the death of the baby.

A content analysis of Australian TV over eighteen months (including some American programmes) revealed that most images of birth were violent and that the woman giving birth was diminished because the action was taken over by a male hero. *Baywatch* screened a labour that lasted less than five minutes. The woman became 'instantly immobilised in ankle deep water and, without removing her swimming suit, delivered the baby on the beach. However, all credit went to the muscle-bound life-saver with his handy little obstetric kit!'[27] Sometimes the heroic action is provided by a female police officer or doctor. In an episode of *Picket Fences*, a woman police officer delivers a breech baby in a car shouting,

'We can do this – I've just got to reach in! Come on – damn it! You can do it! Push, damn it, push!'

In comedy programmes the woman starts to scream at her partner, who also panics, rushing off with the wrong suitcase or the wrong woman. In ER's 'Loves Labor Lost', a mother dies from pre-eclampsia and other complications after being in the emergency room for nine and a half hours and receiving ultrasound, fetal monitoring, an epidural and finally a Caesarean section, but with no attention from either an obstetrician or a midwife.

Talk show topics on Australian TV are startling too: 'Women whose bodies fake pregnancy', 'Birth in strange places', and 'Old age pregnancy'. Presumably to widen the audience, men's emotions, problems and achievements are often centre-stage: 'Gorgeous guys and their babies', and 'Men who hate birth and have not had sex since'.

We have created our own mythology of birth. The drama of this myth is in the medical emergency, the speeding ambulance, the urgent bleep, the staccato calls for assistance, the struggles of a team of doctors and nurses to combat death. There are heart monitors on which the trace flattens out, Caesarean deliveries, massive haemorrhages, resuscitation of the baby. It is a drama that feeds the fears inherent in the medical model of birth and, in this way, further conditions pregnant women to submit to its ritual.

Documentaries on the body's functions put the medical model centre-stage and dramatise what is presented as a conflict between the fetus and the mother. As one (approving) critic comments on the television programme *The Body Story*[28], 'Pregnancy, for example, is explained in terms of a fetal take-over, with the mother to be as a victim of the scheming alien, which first exerts endocrine control over her physiology and then systematically exploits her body for its own interests.'[29]

Reproductive Research

The miracles produced by reproductive research are the new icons of our birth culture. An analysis of stories about fertility treatment published in American women's magazines reveals that 85 per cent of them are a combination of heroic quest, fairy tale and religious miracle.[30] Scientists compete to be the first to discover a technique that makes birth possible to ever more highly unlikely parents: women without ovaries, postmenopausal women, brain-dead women, and men, dead or alive. The Press reports them as stating: 'I make babies.' Their PR photographs show them gleaming with pride, surrounded by attractive children who smile up fondly, lean against them and perch on their knees, or there is a tray-full of chubby babies in front of them. There is something about these photographs, frozen in time, that suggests the Victorian daguerreotype of the family, papa at its centre.

But reproductive experts do not replace only the father. They take over the functions of both father and mother. This is more than patriarchal control. They have displaced both parents. Sex is unnecessary because conception occurs in a petri dish on the lab bench. There is a one in 250 chance of multiple birth with in-vitro fertilisation, and babies are ten times more likely to be born preterm, have twice the risk of spina bifida and heart problems, are forty-seven times more likely to suffer from cerebral palsy – and the risk of death is quadrupled.[31]

Following fertilisation the cell mass is quality controlled and genetically checked. An excess number of fetuses, or imperfect ones, are sucked out and selectively aborted. Ultimately, the remaining products of conception can be delivered by Caesarean section, with everything under scientific control.

Our magicians and miracle makers are the scientists who make it possible for a woman to bear eight babies, to produce babies after the menopause, or with another woman's ovum and sperm from a bank. These scientists open up new possibilities in reproduction in the search to eradicate genetic disease and disability, and to perfect human beings. In doing so, they seek to demonstrate the superiority of the scientific over the natural. We are told that advances in in-vitro fertilisation, for example, have upped success rates for infertile women to almost twice that achieved by natural conception. Figures from the British Human Fertilisation and Embryology Authority show that some clinics achieve live-birth rates of up to 40 per cent for each attempt, compared with only 20 to 25 per cent a month with sexual intercourse.[32]

The Merlin-like charisma of reproductive scientists is reinforced by the media in shock headlines: 'Test Tube Success Rivals Natural Birth' and 'Embryo Created From Four Animals'. The latter introduced a story about the fusing of the cells of four different animal species – a sheep, a pig, a rat and a rhesus macaque monkey – with a cow's ovum which had its own nucleus removed, with the prospect of the development of human embryos within cows' ova. These ova will serve as early incubators and produce embryos that can be used for therapeutic cloning. The research scientist is reported as saying, 'If we can do it with rhesus macaque monkeys there is no reason to suppose we cannot do it with human cells.' A colleague adds, 'We showed that the embryo implanted and the pregnancy lasted for about thirty days but we could not recover the foetus.'[33] Reproductive medicine has propelled us into scientific Odyssey and a new world of experiment to which our old value systems are ill-adapted and which leaves us feeling helpless in the face of forces beyond our control.

The anthropologist Levi-Strauss claimed that the West is culturally impoverished. Traditionally, birth and death are ripe with meanings that penetrate the whole of social life, but we have emptied both these experiences of everything that is not merely physiological. Women's bodies are managed in pregnancy and childbirth as if they were machines always at risk of breaking down, in much the same way that a car is checked and repaired and the engine revved up by a mechanic. This might work if women were machines. But in mammals, and especially in human beings, all physical functions are affected by what is going on in our minds. Breathing, digestion, elimination of waste, heart rate and blood pressure, and in labour uterine function, are profoundly affected by emotions, beliefs and relationships. It has been known for a long time that stress can make labour slow down or stop altogether, and cause uterine inco-ordination and excessive pain.[34]

We still have much to learn about the effects of stress, and how mind and body interact, in pregnancy and birth.

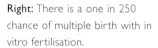

Right: There is a one in 250 chance of multiple birth with in vitro fertilisation.

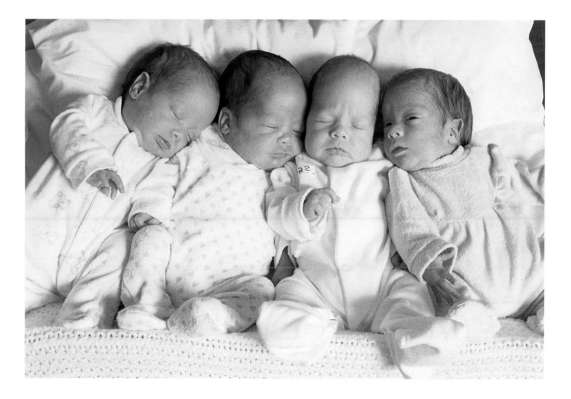

Chapter 3

Birth and Spirit

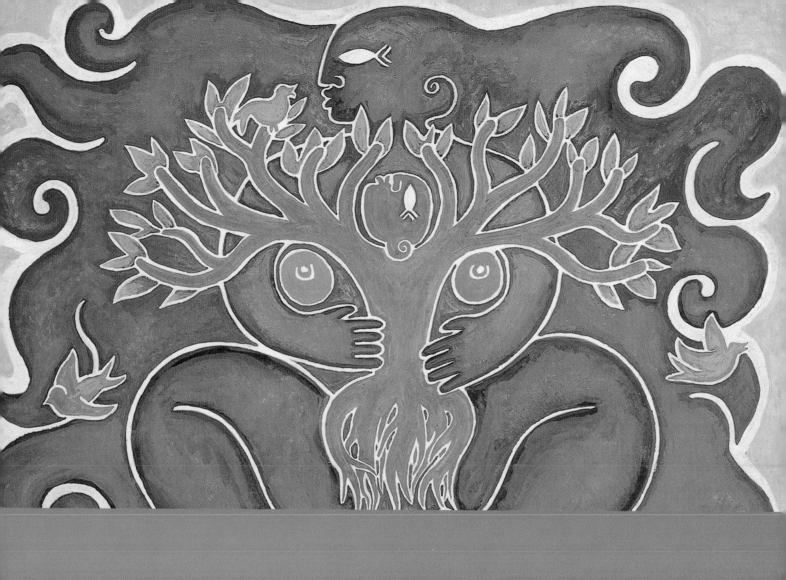

From prehistory on, birth, coming into life, like death, going out of it, has been a spiritual matter. It has been shaped by myth and magic, patterned by ritual, infused with hope and longing and expressed through sacred acts. Birth was the domain of the Great Mother Goddess, the giver of all life.

As medicine took over birth, and saved lives, the Mother Goddess faded. Ritual practices were fragmented and became 'old wives' tales'. They are the almost forgotten shreds of a previously strong belief system about women, blood, birth and breastmilk.

Right: Three terracotta fertility goddesses from the beginning of the third millennium BC.

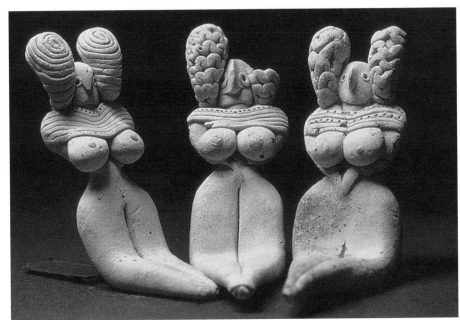

India

She who carries the universe in her womb,
source of all creative energy,
Maha Devi who conceives
and bears and nourishes
all that exists.[1]

Navajo, North America

In the beginning nothing existed except Spider Woman, she who was called Sussistanako, Thinking Woman, Thought Woman. In the dark purple light that glowed at the Dawn of Being, Spider Woman spun a fine thread from east to west, from north to south . . . and then she sat by those threads that stretched to the four horizons, and sang in a voice that was deep and sweet, and as she sang, she gave birth to two daughters, Ut Set, who was the mother of the Pueblo people, and Nau Ut Set, the mother of all other beings.[2]

Tao Te Ching

It is named the Mysterious Female.
And the Doorway of the Mysterious Female is the base from which Heaven and Earth sprang.
It is there within us all the while.[3]

Sumer

Ama Tu An Ki,
mother who gave birth
to heaven and earth
first creator of the universe
who shapes the whole of life
and controls the fate of each one –
most ancient of all.[4]

Tiamat (Babylonian)

When heaven above had not yet been named
Nor the earth beneath,
There was Tiamat herself, she who gave birth to all.
The waters were mingled.
No pasture land had yet been formed,
Nor was there even a reed marsh to be seen.[5]

Shapes scratched in rock, perhaps once drawn in sand or earth, forms modelled in clay; these are evidence of the intense spirituality of the process of bringing new life into the world.

The earliest surviving representations of the goddess, from the Palaeolithic, are well-rounded figures with huge breasts and buttocks and exaggerated sexual organs. They often have no heads, since these are relatively unimportant. The goddess may be great with child, but there is rarely a baby in her arms.

In the Neolithic, a goddess holding a baby appears, together with a totally different icon, a purely abstract figure, consisting of geometric lines.

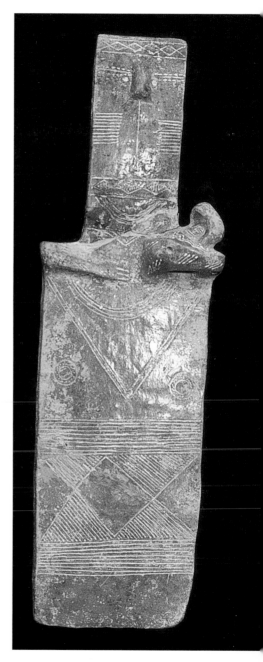

Above: Goddess with child. A red terracotta idol, dating from the second millennium BC.

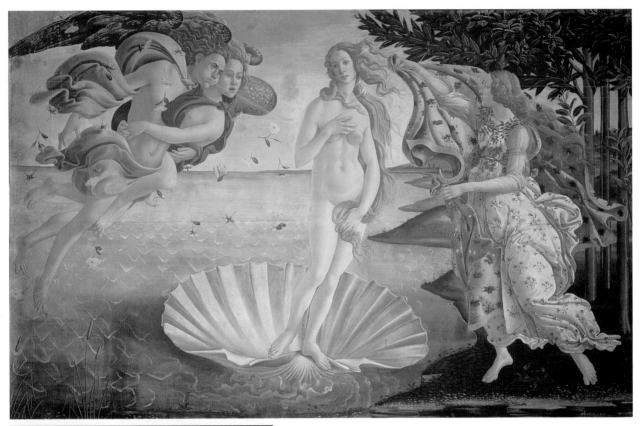

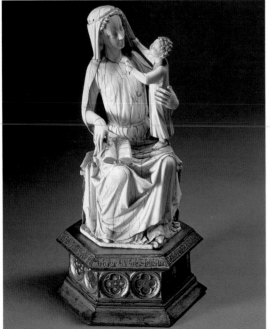

Later still, the son of the goddess becomes the divine Son, and in the historical era the Son has deposed the Mother, who is in the background as the Mother of God. She is no longer a sexual being. She is Venus rising from the waves, or Mary with child.

Above: 'The Birth of Venus' by Botticelli, the goddess no longer a mother, but maiden.

Left: A 13th-century ivory sculpture of the Virgin and child. The power of the goddess has been replaced by the tenderness of the Mother of God.

The Birth Symbol

In many different cultures, from the Palaeolithic on, human fertility is a powerful force that causes crops to grow, fish and animals to be caught in the hunt, domesticated animals to bear young, and the whole society to flourish. There is an element in childbirth that is sacramental. An ikat from the island of Mindanao in the Philippines tells the story of how human fertility and the abundance of nature are linked. When women are pregnant the soil is bare. When women give birth, the gardens flourish.

Since time immemorial, the concept of the fertile womb and the life-giving vagina has been an important symbolic element in weaving, pottery and other crafts created by women. It is the counterpart of the phallic symbol, and has been largely ignored by men.

One widespread birth symbol is a diamond with hooked arms and legs. It first appears 8,000 years ago and is 'our oldest surviving religious image'.[6] Throughout the Middle East and North Africa, the Western Pacific and large parts of Asia and South America, this hooked diamond can be found in rugs and wall hangings made by women. At first sight it is purely abstract. But in some of its forms, and if you look more closely, it becomes a standing woman with legs and arms bent. The baby is often shown as a cross in the middle of the diamond.

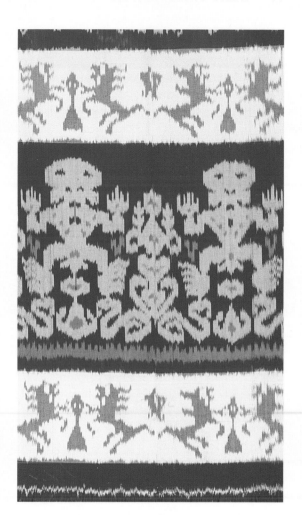

Above: An ikat wall hanging with a woman giving birth, showing the hooked arms and legs of the birth symbol.

Most powerful birth images have been made in materials which decay rapidly – woven fabrics, for example. But pottery images have survived, usually in fragments. A hooked diamond appears on a pot made 6,000 years ago in central Turkey, at Catal Huyuk in Anatolia, where from the Neolithic onwards the worship of the Great Mother Goddess produced a rich treasure of pots, sculpture and paintings, and where the Greek goddesses of fertility were born.

Hesiod (c750BC)

First the Voice came into being. Then the heavy breasted Earth, the enduring home of all.

Out of Night came Light and Day, children conceived by union in love with Darkness.

Then Earth gave birth to the Sky and it covered her entirely.

She created great mountains, the beautiful places where the gods dwell.

And great stretches of sea in its foaming rage.

From her union with Sky the ocean was born.

She gave birth, too, to the violent Cyclopes and made the thunder and the lightning bolt.

A single eye stood in the centre of their foreheads and strength and power and skill were in their hands.

As each was about to be born the Sky would not let them reach the light of day.

Earth felt the strain within her and groaned.

Then Sky came to her drawing the night behind him.

He lay on top of Earth and stretched above her . . .

*And his son Cronus reached out with a sickle and cut off his father's penis and
    testicles and threw them away.*

The blood that spurted from them entered Mother Earth.

In the course of time she gave birth to the Spirits of Vengeance.

And the sea white foam flowed from the divine flesh.

And in the foam a girl began to grow.

She floated towards Holy Cythera.

Then reached Cyprus.

And stepped out, a Goddess, tender and beautiful.

And round her slender feet the grass shot up.

*She is called Aphrodite by gods and men because she grew
    in the foam of the sea.*[7]

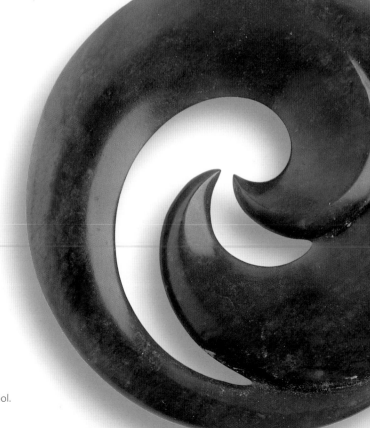

Right: A greenstone Maori
pendant; an abstract
representation of the fern,
which is a Maori birth symbol.

The hooked diamond symbol is a common symbol in carpets and kilims throughout North Africa. These are woven by women, though sold by men. Men cannot 'see' the birth image that is sacred to women. Carpet-dealers in Morocco, eager to explain the meaning of symbols in the rugs they sell, speak with authority and conviction about most of them. But when I enquired about the meaning of the hooked diamond they paused, looked perplexed, and then suggested 'men at prayer', 'a two-humped camel', or 'the mosque'. They saw these shapes with men's eyes.

The hooked diamond may have been a code in the symbolic language of weaving that was special to women, a cabalistic symbol of birth-giving power. 'A secret sign – a membership card, so to speak – used by members of the early (Christian) church, for identification was the sign of the fish . . . The birth symbol, embroidered on the bag carried by a midwife, may once have served a similar purpose: a sign of shared belief, incomprehensible to the uninitiated'.[8]

The teardrop or 'boteh' is a birth symbol in Kashmir. It was taken over by Scottish merchants, incorporated into shawls manufactured in Paisley in the 17th century, and appears in the paisley patterns seen in furniture fabric, dress materials and scarves. It is a theme reiterated in Persian carpets. Although it looks like a teardrop, it represents the Tree of Life, a fertility image which dates from the Babylonian era.

Creation

Childbirth takes place at the intersection of time; in all cultures it links past, present and future. In traditional cultures birth unites the world of 'now' with the world of the ancestors, and is part of the great tree of life extending in time and eternity. A central theme of all religions is the emergence of human beings (often in the form of monsters, serpents or mystical creatures), of birth to a male god, or the splitting of a single animal in two. But birth goddesses are the oldest divinities of all.

The Mexican goddess Coatlicue dwelt on a mountain peak inside a cloud. There she gave birth to the moon, the sun and the other gods. She was the mother of all things.

Panama

In the days before the world began, Mu gave birth to the sun, and taking the sun as her lover she gave birth to the moon. She mated with her grandson Moon and brought forth the stars, so many that they filled the heavens. Then she mated with the stars and her sacred womb once again stirred with life, and thus Mu brought forth all the animals and plants.[9]

The Great Mother Goddess often breathes life into clay figures or other objects modelled by the divine hands, harnessing all the powers of nature to help in that work.

Babylon

Aruru, most ancient of all,
creator of Life,
Mami, divine mother of all,
womb that gave birth to all humanity
and to this day creates our destiny . . .
it was she who made all life
by pinching off 14 pieces of clay
and placing a brick between them.
She made 7 women
whom she placed on the left.
She made 7 men
whom she placed on the right.
Shaping them into people
she then put them on the earth.[10]

Ancient China

To the valleys of the wide flowing Hwang Ho came
the goddess Nu Kwa and there from the rich gold
earth she fashioned the race of golden beings,
carefully working the features of each with skilful
fingers, the ancestors of the Chinese people.[11]

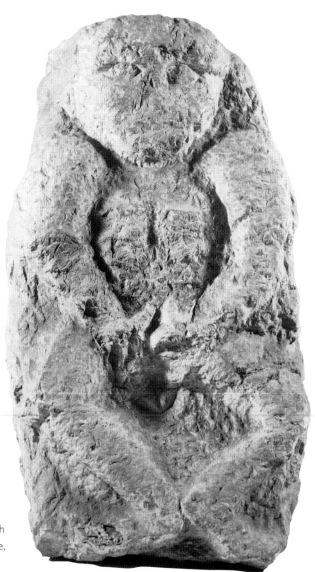

Right: A rock carving of a birth goddess found at Carne Castle, County Westmeath, Ireland.

Creation myths express wonder and astonishment at life coming out of nothing, and often, too, the pain of that transformation and the festive delight of creation. Birth goddesses embody sacramental beliefs about human birth.

Prehistoric birth scenes were carved on rock in cave shrines. When women depict the act of birth-giving in pottery they illustrate not only human women but the great elemental force of life-giving power, the goddess who moves heaven and earth in her birth pangs, giving birth to mountains, rivers and seas, and to all created things.

Greece

Her black wings furled over her nest,
Nikta gave birth to the egg in the wind,
the egg from which desire
entered the world at the beginning of time,
so that humanity could come to being.[12]

Below: A Boeotian goddess with fish womb, animals and birds, from the 8th century BC.

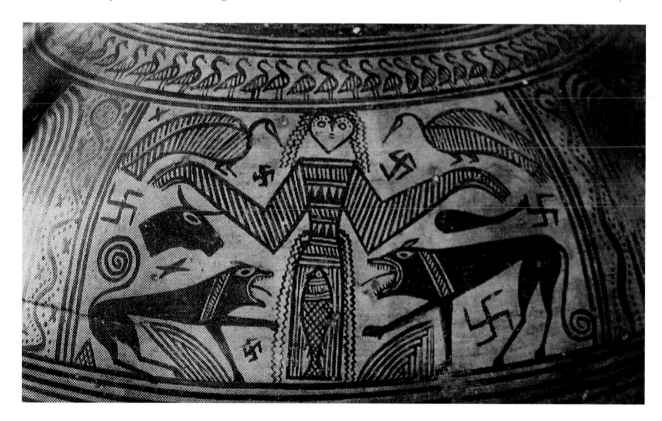

With the beginnings of agriculture in the Neolithic, the birth goddess became a goddess of the sowing of seed and of the harvest. In Greece, an ear of wheat was the symbol of Eleusis, where the mysteries in honour of Goddess Demeter, or Ceres the Corn Mother, were enacted. The central drama of this was a sacred marriage and the birth of a holy child. Corn dollies made at the time of harvest well into the 20th century, and still to be found in craft shops, were a symbol of birth and rebirth.

Religions in Conflict

In the Iron Age, the birth goddess disappeared from view as warrior tribes swept through Europe and the countries of the Near East, bringing with them a patriarchal religion. The religions they superimposed on the old goddess faith entailed worship of a male god, but women continued to revere the goddess and turned to her in childbirth. Goddess worship became a domestic religion, one in which women came together to celebrate rites that sustained the family and supported them in the great transitions of their lives, while state religion and the religious institutions in which men were involved became dominant.

The idols that Christian rulers and religious leaders later ordered to be destroyed were invariably those of goddesses and the symbols of their power. The Muslim faith equally condemned the religions of goddesses. The Koran explicitly states: 'Allah will not tolerate idolatry. The pagans pray to females.'

Three great goddesses survived the initial onslaught of patriarchal religion: Ishtar of Sumeria, Isis of Egypt, and Cybele of Anatolia. Ishtar, Inanna in southern Sumeria, was Queen of Heaven and Earth, First Daughter of the Moon and Opener of the Womb. Her symbol was an inverted horse-shoe shape which represented both the uterus and the sheep fold and byre in which lambs and calves were born. Isis was worshipped not only in Egypt but in Greece and, with Roman colonisation of a large part of Europe, as far as the Danube and the Rhine. She manifested herself in many forms: as a cow goddess who gave milk to her people, as a sow, a bird, the Tree of Life, and the mother of the baby Horus. In classical Greece, Artemis, the Goddess of the Hunt, was also the Goddess of Childbirth. A chorus in a play by Euripides sang: 'Once I felt this thrill of pain in my womb, I cried out for Artemis in heaven, who loves the hunt and whose care relieves those giving birth. She came to me then and eased me.'

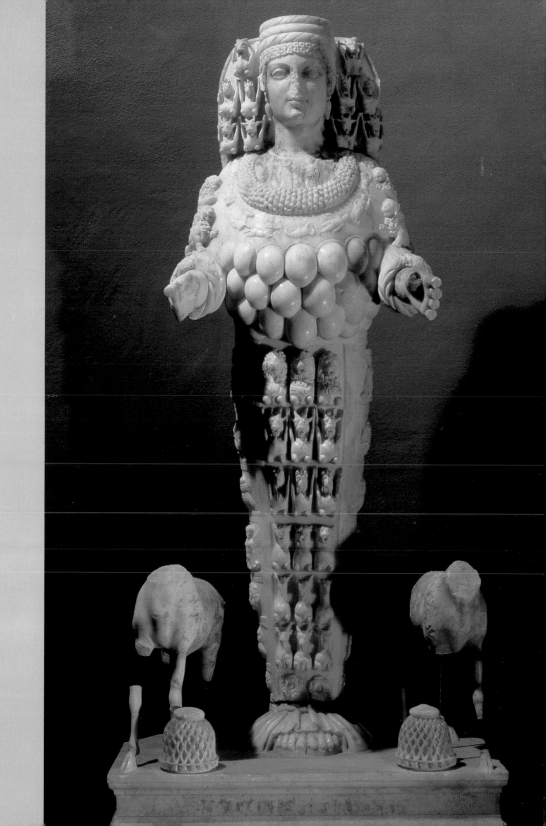

Left: Ishtar, Goddess of Fertility; c. 2000BC.

Right: A marble statue of Artemis, Goddess of Fertility, from the 2nd century AD.

Manifestations of the Goddess

The Goddess Artemis, whose worship evolved in Anatolia, was a manifestation of Cybele, and later, with the coming of Christianity, she metamorphosed into Mary, the Mother of God. The mother with a child in her lap, often suckling it, is variously Isis, Cybele, Artemis – and Mary.

Christmas was originally celebrated on 6 January – Epiphany. This was the festival in Egypt of the birth of a son to the Greek Kore, whose other name was 'the Maiden', who in turn evolved from Isis. She was also known as Nut or Neit, and Hathor. With every sunrise, worshippers could see in the sky the blood of her birth-giving. As patriarchal religion took over, the dawn was seen in a different way; it was the blood of the serpent of darkness who had been killed by the sun. But Nut, or Neit, remained as Goddess of the Night Sky and the Darkness.

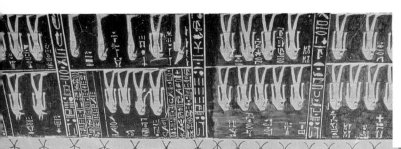

The Goddess Neit, Egypt

The earth nestles between Her thighs.
Daily She gives birth to the Sun,
each evening accepting him back into Her body
just as each mortal returns unto Her
when the span of life is over.[13]

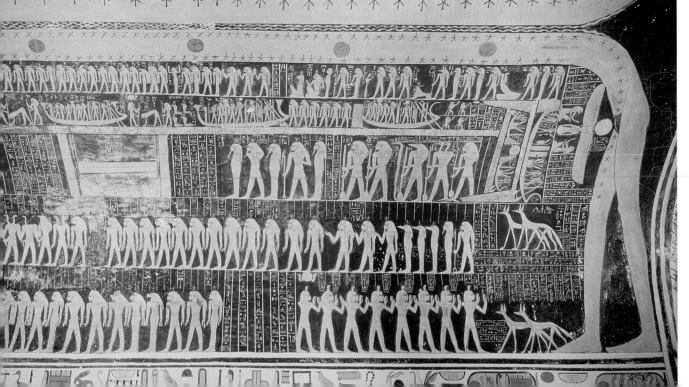

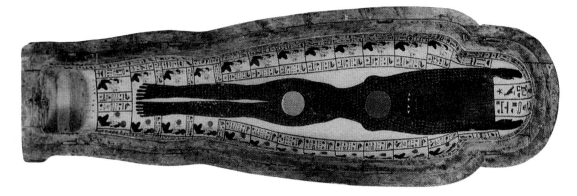

Right: A sarcophagus as the womb of the Goddess Nut. The soul of the dead person enters her body and emerges to be reborn like the sun. 7th century BC.

She was depicted in coffins, on both the base and the lid, as the mother holding the dead body so that it could be reborn like the sun.

In all religions birth goddesses merge with each other, take on fresh forms and new characteristics as the religions evolve. Not only were the goddesses of Greece transformed into the Mary of Christianity, but the most ancient Mother Goddess of them all found a place in the Gnostic gospels. These gospels were eradicated from the New Testament by the year 200AD, but until then Gnostic Christians referred to God as both 'the Mother', creator of all, and as Sophia, or wisdom. She was the goddess who existed before anything else came into being.

In every culture, goddesses, though worshipped as goddesses of the hunt, for example, or devil goddesses fighting against the power of the gods of patriarchal religion, incorporate concepts of birth. The birth goddess is the mother of all life. She is depicted in rock drawings and in fired clay as a woman with enormous breasts, her body swollen with many pregnancies. Sometimes in these cave paintings and lithographs, and in patterns on pots, a simple triangle represents the goddess. It is an abstract symbol of her vagina, the entrance to her uterus.

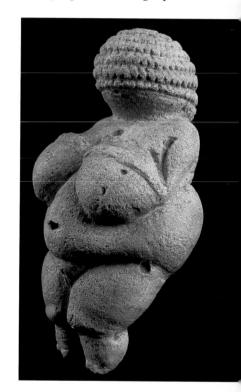

Left: An Egyptian wall painting from the 11th century BC, showing the day and night journey of the sun. The Goddess Nut swallows the sun at night and gives birth to it again each morning.

Right: A limestone and chalk statue of the fertility goddess often called the 'Venus of Willendorf'; c. 20000BC.

A bird goddess was worshipped throughout Europe and in North Africa in Palaeolithic times. She laid the egg of the universe, from which, as it cracked open, all life emerged. She has a long neck and her body is ovoid. Sometimes she takes the form of a vase, which becomes an image of the uterus, with curving lines to represent life-giving water. In northern Greece there is a creation myth in which Eurynome rises out of Chaos and dances the sea and sky into being. Then she seizes the north wind and moulds it in her hands to become a great serpent which makes her pregnant with all life. She is transformed into a dove and lays an egg on the waters. The serpent coils round it and it hatches to give birth to the whole of nature and human beings.

The Minoan and Mycenaean bird goddesses in Crete had human faces. They evolved into the goddesses of Greece. In the *Odyssey*, Athene is able to turn into six kinds of bird: 'Athene of the flashing eyes disappeared flying up into the air, like a bird', and later, 'darted up and perched on the smoky roof-beam of the hall, in the actual form of a swallow'.[14]

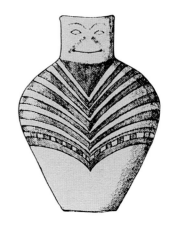

Above: A bird goddess vase. Chevrons symbolising wings decorate the body of the vase; c. 5300–5000BC.

Egypt

The Lady of Flame,
The Lady of Flaming Waters
The Lady who shed Her skin
to be born again and again and again,
for Ua Zit had existed before Egypt was born,
and before the Creation.[15]

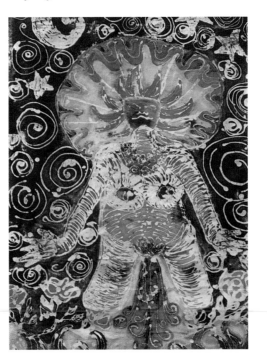

Left:
'The giant wave rises to a peak
breath-stopping
and the world splits open.

Waters flow
and on their salt flood a child
presses deep, stinging sweet
and urgent for birth.'

Sheila Kitzinger,
A Celebration of Birth.[16]

In the Neolithic, the goddess became Mistress of the Upper Waters. Just as the waters break before a child is born, so rain pours from the sky and gushes to water plants and quench the thirst of animals and human beings. The Goddess of the Lower Waters was often a serpent. She coiled and slithered like the rivers and their tributaries that snaked across the earth.

The Goddess Nammu of Sumerian mythology is a snake who gave birth to heaven and earth. This, in turn, is linked to the labyrinths and coiling, meandering shapes that also represent birth. Today women in childbirth sometimes find a similar winding, spiralling shape, perhaps produced by a computer drawing, a helpful visual focus in childbirth.

In Slav mythology, the Sky Woman is derived from the birth goddess. She brings the water that will ensure a good harvest.[17] In the past it was believed that she had sexual intercourse with the thunder god in early summer, and there was a great festival at that time. The Goddess of Water is essentially a birth goddess, and in parts of Russia young women prayed to 'the little mother', Matushka, on 1 October, a Greek Orthodox holy day, that they might find a man and get pregnant. Greek Orthodox priests forbade these 'rusalka' rites, which included dancing, singing, throwing leaves into water, and sexual abandon, but they continued to be celebrated in May and June until the 20th century.

Birth goddesses are also usually goddesses of the moon. They control the swing of tides, the changing seasons and the phases of the menstrual cycle. In the rhythm of the goddess's waning and waxing, nature dies and is reborn, just as the shape of the moon is constantly changing. While the sun is usually perceived as male, the moon is female, and has her own powerful mythology that incorporates death as well as birth.

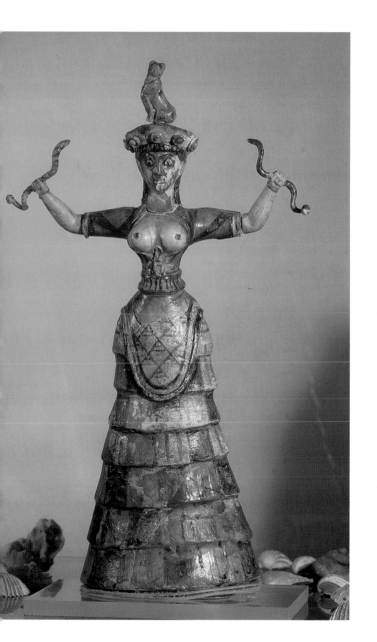

Left: A Minoan Snake Goddess, dating from the 17th century BC.

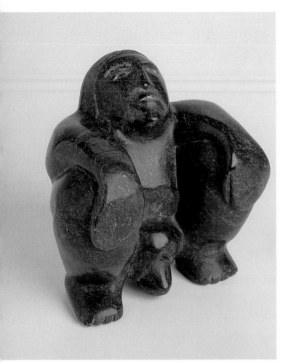

In Mexico representations of the Aztec Goddess of Birth do not just show an individual woman giving birth; they embody the energy of all women and the strength of the goddess who helps each woman in childbirth and to whom the midwife prays for a safe delivery. The same power is evident in a contemporary Inuit sculpture of birth-giving.

Goddesses protect dangerous passages in the life of the individual and the community. The Japanese Birth Goddess Ubagami (or Obagami) is the Goddess of Boundaries and helps people across them. She calls the spirit of the baby into the world of human beings. In villages around Lake Inawashiro, Ubagami shrines stand on the boundary lines between two areas, two villages, or two parts of a village. In human life it is this goddess who guards the threshold between life and death.

As we have seen, the wearing of the *hara obi*, or birth sash, is a religious rite that remains an integral part of the ceremony surrounding pregnancy and birth in modern Japan. In accounts of birth in noble families dating from the Heian era (794–1192), there are descriptions of how the *obi* was used. At that time it was always of white silk and was put on by the father of the baby on an auspicious day chosen by a diviner, who also selected the place where the birth hut should be built. The father built the hut and in it was placed an amulet and inscribed prayer for a safe and easy birth. During labour the diviner and the priest prayed for a good outcome, while the attending women plucked bow strings to make a humming sound that drove away all evil.

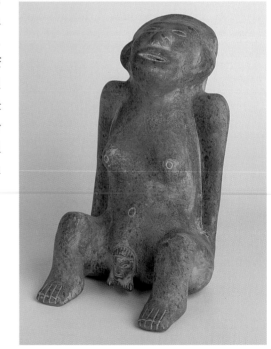

Above left: A modern Inuit soapstone carving of a woman giving birth.

Right: A Mexican terracotta sculpture of birth-giving.

In modern Japan the baby's paternal grandmother presents the *obi*, and she and her daughter-in-law visit the shrine together to bless the pregnancy and pray for a good birth. Photographs of this visit to the shrine are found in many Japanese families' photograph albums. When a woman visits the shrine she also gets a talisman, a small brocade bag with a slip of paper inside it on which are written the words 'Easy birth'.

Special shrines are dedicated to the *obi*, but it is available from any shrine. It is a bleached cotton sash about three metres long which the pregnant woman puts on during the Dog Day because the dog gives birth to its puppies easily. When worn during labour it helps ease birth. It is also a divine messenger that can chase away evil and guide the baby out. The child's spirit comes from the mother's family, so this sash is usually given by the woman's mother-in-law. In some parts of Japan the cast skin of a snake was used in the past as an *obi*, symbolising rebirth.

The Tree of Life

The birth goddess is still revered and offerings made to her in many traditional cultures. She is the goddess of the ancestral line, goddess of all our pasts, and dates back to the roots of humanity. She is also the goddess of nature, of earth, sea, the wind, the moon, the rain and the stars, and of all beasts and birds. In Hawaii she is known by two names, and manifests herself in two different ways. Papa is Mother Earth, the original female principle; Pele is the 'Grandmother' – or Tutu – and appears in dreams in the guise of an old woman.[18]

Outside the parish church of St Martins in Guernsey there is a granite figure of a birth goddess from 1,000 years BC. She, too, is the Grandmother, la Granmère du Chimpière.

Traditionally in South America, the midwife has a pottery pipe in the form of the figure of a birthing woman, on which she blows to summon the blessing spirits to come to help and protect the labouring woman and her baby.

Right: In Guatemala, Peru and Mexico birth pipes summoned the blessing spirits during labour.

Among the Ibo of Nigeria it is believed that each newborn child comes from a community of unborn spirit babies with whom it has been playing. When a baby cries or smiles unexpectedly it is communicating with these spirit babies and trying to persuade them to join the human family, but they are urging it to return to them.[19]

The oneness of human birth and the rest of creation, the unity of human life with nature, is characteristic of beliefs surrounding pregnancy and birth in Eastern cultures. In Malaysia it is believed that before conception takes place the father has already been pregnant in his brain for 40 days. The baby descends from his brain to his penis, and from there enters the woman's uterus. It is like a seed planted in the earth and grows like a flower inside the mother's body. The world is formed from four elements – earth, air, fire, water – and when semen is added they create a baby.[20]

On the island of Bali the journey through life is suffused with religious ceremony. The world is divided by four compass points, and for each point there is a god. Every day there are rituals to observe. Birth is shaped by ritual, too. The baby is born with four 'brothers' who guard its life: the amniotic fluid, the birth blood, the umbilical cord, and the placenta. 'Ari-ari', the placenta, is the most powerful brother of all.

The first brother, the amniotic fluid, comes from the God of East and West. The second, the blood, from Brahma, and soil red with blood is taken up as a votive offering to Brahma. The third is the cord, which is related to the ancestors and the setting sun, and this is placed in a small box and hung from a necklace that the baby wears in order to ward off danger. The placenta is Lord of the Graveyard, protecting the bodies of the dead and guarding the living from illness. It is ritually placed in half a coconut that has been lined with leaves and pebbles. The two halves of the shell are closed and bound up by the baby's father while a prayer is recited. He erects a small shrine over the burial place of the placenta and the family make offerings every day to the baby's 'brothers'. In this way the child is linked to and protected by the ancestors and by the sun at its setting every evening throughout its life.[21]

The Midwife's Spiritual Role

Traditionally, the midwife is not merely a birth attendant with special expertise. She has a spiritual function in helping the baby to birth, the woman to become a mother, and in creating the setting for birth and the time immediately following it so that it is right for this spiritual transition. In many birth cultures she is also responsible for prayers, chants, invocations and other actions to clear the way for birth and to nurture the right relationships between all those participating.

Traditional midwives in the Philippines, the *hilots*, combine practical and supernatural skills, guided by the spirits of ancestors who were 'gifted' in the same way. A World Health Organisation (WHO) report states that they are revered in their communities. They know how to dispose of the placenta so that evil spirits cannot find it, and, since 'the gate of Heaven' is open for forty-four days after childbirth, attend the mother throughout this time to massage and bind her abdomen, as well as helping with the housework and other children.[22]

Similarly, midwives in Malaysia can deal with evil spirits and prevent them attacking the mother and baby. The *bidan* understand the rites that must be enacted to purify the woman and make her less vulnerable to these spirits, the positions which she should adopt to avoid them, and how to make the house safe with the leaves of prickly pandanus and charms to bar their way.[23]

The Indian *dai*, usually perceived as an ignorant 'traditional birth attendant', only useful as a stop-gap until women can have proper medical attention but who can be taught to transfer messages about contraception and nutrition to the poor women whom she attends, is a shamanistic practitioner and specialist in religious ritual. She

Traditionally, the midwife is not merely a birth attendant with special expertise. She has a spiritual function in helping the baby to birth, the woman to become a mother, and in creating the setting for birth and the time immediately following it so that it is right for this spiritual transition.

is an 'experiential guide to the labouring woman, using such tools as altered states of consciousness, spirit guides and sympathetic magic'.[24]

Almost everywhere, the religious work done by the midwife is distinct from the dominant, male-directed religion of the wider culture. It is part of the religion of women, and as such is treated with contempt or amused tolerance by male specialists.

The midwife works at the intersection of time, as generation gives way to generation. In helping to make the birth space, she creates a place of sanctuary. She is a shepherdess between the two worlds of the spiritual and human, and her skills lie at the point where the emotional and the biological touch each other and interact. She tends the tree of life. In an exhibition of West African coffins the organisers explained why this array of brightly coloured, gaudy, exuberant coffins in the shape of animals, birds, fish, cars and houses were significant: 'Millions of people are no longer able to see their life as a link in the chain of hundreds of generations, as the African and Asian cultures do, or used to do. Making the individual time dimension absolute makes people vulnerable in relation to death, and with it, to past and future. One's relationship to the past inevitably determines the relationship to the future. The way a culture, or more specifically a family, views parents, grandparents and its own traditions, determines its ideas about the future.'

The increasing absence of concrete traditions and of any historic consciousness means that millions of children in the urbanised world lack a consciousness of 'the succession of the generations'.

In much the same way, when birth is perceived as part of a greater tree of life, extending in time and eternity, and a link with the ancestors, it has a deeper meaning for the individual, and for society. A significant part of the traditional midwife's role is to acknowledge that meaning and to empower the mother with the spiritual strength that comes from the ancestors.

In many traditional societies illness is believed to result from disharmony. To heal is to restore harmony between hot and cold humours, between male and female principles, or Yin and Yang. It is the midwife's task to create harmony between the mother and her body, the family and the ancestors, and the family and the wider community. For birth to go well relationships must be right. She may advise offering a gift to someone who has been wronged. In peasant Greece, anyone who has quarrelled with the woman giving birth must seek her forgiveness so that harmony surrounds the birth. They come to her begging formal pardon by offering her water to drink from their cupped hands. In the former Yugoslavia, Jewish women gave alms to the poor when their labour started.

Sometimes midwives use the image of a flower, one which opens as the cervix dilates, to help a woman to focus on the opening of her body. It is a common practice in southern India, Malaysia and in rural parts of Mediterranean countries such as southern Italy and Greece. The birth flower is the rose of Jericho. Apparently dry and shrivelled, it is placed beside the mother and gradually spreads wide all its petals in the heat of the birth room. It is an intense visual image. In the Christian tradition the same flower is known in Italy as 'the rose of Mary'. In Greece it is 'the hand of the Mother of God'. For the labouring woman it is as if Mary labours with her, her hand spreading wide all the petals of the cervix so that the child may be born.

Prayer is one way of creating and sustaining harmony with spiritual forces. In Hawaii, the midwife was called Kahuna Pale Keiki and was also a priest. After praying to the Goddess of Childbirth, she could take away the mother's pain and transfer it from her to anyone she chose. In many cultures there are special birth prayers and invocations. In both the Jewish and Muslim faith, for example, there are birth prayers to be recited by the father while his wife labours, and others to celebrate the baby's birth.

The birth flower is the rose of Jericho. Apparently dry and shrivelled, it is placed beside the mother and gradually spreads wide all its petals in the heat of the birth room. It is an intense visual image.

The spiritual nature of birth is central to Christianity. Mary's pregnancy is of God, not man. Like many of the goddesses before her, she is a virgin. She gives birth in a stable surrounded by animals, a scene in which there is an echo of the goddesses Cybele and Artemis.

Like the birth goddesses before her, the Virgin Mary protected women in childbirth. In the 16th century, Catholic women in England wore a special sash, the girdle of Mary, in pregnancy and birth, or a woman in labour might have worn her own girdle once it had been wrapped around a sanctified bell. With the dissolution of the monasteries in 1536, holy girdles, belts and necklaces that had been lent out to women in labour were discovered. Reformist churchmen tried to suppress these ritual practices, but in the intimacy of the birth room they continued. However, midwives had to swear on oath to avoid 'any kind of sorcery or incarnation'.[25]

The holy sacrament was considered the strongest medicine of all. A 17th-century prayer in a French book, 'Dévotions particulières pour les femmes enceintes', reads: 'Oh Mother of the holiest one of holies who approached nearest to His divine perfection and so became mother to such a son, obtain for me by your Grace . . . the favour to let me suffer with patience the pain that overwhelms me and let me be delivered from this ill. Have compassion upon me. I cannot hold out without your help.'[26]

Birth has always been considered a testing time for women, entailing courage and endurance. In Englishwomen's diaries and letters of the 17th and 18th centuries, it was perceived as a spiritual journey and a transforming experience, as well as a physiological process.

A mother emerged triumphant from labour, rather like a warrior returning victorious from battle. Women wrote of the pain of travail. But the experience of birth was much larger than this. It was a drama in which there was a sense of unity, both with other living things and with a long line of women in the past.

In a very different culture, women of the tribal people in the Kalahari desert of Botswana and Namibia in southern Africa are exceptional in that with their second and subsequent births they do not expect help from other women during birth. Yet they, too, see birth as a transforming experience which draws on spiritual energy. They are proud of giving birth out of doors, in the bush, alone. While men dare death by going into trances and hunting antelope, women accept responsibility for birth. They believe that the only enemy is fear. Women aim to enter 'a powerful altered state of consciousness, one in which great learning and personal growth are possible'.[27] The solitary birth experience is seen as an important process in maturation, in becoming an adult able to be powerful, responsive and productive.

Birth Mysteries

In Tudor and Stuart England, the practices surrounding childbirth were kept largely secret from men. Yet almost everything we learn about birth at that time was written by men. Though the established Church tried to control childbirth, it was not very successful in doing so. The rites that women enacted resembled those of an underground religion in which men were permitted no part. As a result, it is a 'through the keyhole' view of birth. According to Church doctrine, the birth of a baby was at once evidence of the curse of Eve and the grace of God. It was a strange mix of sin, redemption and blessing. Aristocratic women expressed themselves in this language of the Church in their diaries and letters.

Through the 16th and 17th centuries, 'The Christian Church, predominantly a male institution, provided the language and told the stories that governed thinking about human reproduction. But the extent to which the public Christian discourse on childbirth was echoed within the private womanly domain of the birth room is something we may never know . . . Motherhood, from the pulpit perspective, recapitulated the entire spiritual history of humankind. The woman bore children and suffered because she was stained by original sin. Yet miraculously, through Christ's redemption, she could be saved. Childbirth involved sorrow, shame and chastisement; yet under Christ the woman's labour was part of a covenant of sanctification, mercy and eternal comfort.'

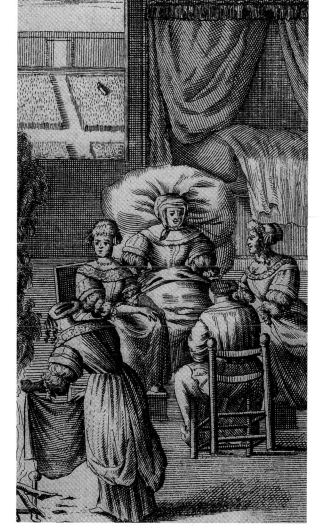

Right: A woodcut of a woman in labour with her god-sibs and midwife. From *The Ten Pleasures of Marriage*, 1682.

Sermons, prayers and pious meditations reiterated this theme in countless dispositions on childbearing in Elizabethan and Stuart England.[28] The Stuart minister, John Ward, tells of how, when a country woman was in labour, Lady Puckering was sent for to help: 'When she came she exhorted her to patience, and told her that this misery was brought upon her sex by her grandmother Eve, by eating an apple. "Was it?" said she, "I wish the apple had choked her." Whereupon my lady was constrained to turn herself about, and go out of the room and laugh.'[29]

Midwives were supposed to be licensed by the Church, but many worked with no such authorisation. 'The female subculture of childbirth included intimate practices and beliefs that were barely suspected by husbands or priests, were long resistant to reform, and which remain virtually inaccessible to historians.'[30] Even midwives who were licensed were suspected of using 'superstitious ceremonies, orisons, charms or devilish rites or sorceries', according to Bishop Barnes of Durham, who instructed his clergy in 1577 to discipline these midwives, and ordered them to be put on oath not to 'use any kind of sorcery or incantation'.[31] When labour was difficult it was common practice for a passage from the Bible to be written on a piece of paper which was soaked in water; the woman then drank the water. These charms were also lode-stones and eagle stones. Lode-stones were precious or semi-precious stones – quartz, sapphire, agate, jasper, coral or amber – that a woman wore during pregnancy to prevent miscarriage or premature birth, and also during labour to ease birth. They were a link to the power of the earth and ancient times when God formed the rocks. An eagle stone is a stone inside a stone, symbolic of a baby inside the mother's body. It has this name because it was supposed to be found in eagles' nests. It drew on a sense of harmony with nature, mother and baby nestled together like the stone within the stone, and perhaps also linked with the strength of birds that can fly over great hills. In 1658 an aristocratic woman who wore an eagle stone at her neck during pregnancy had a very slow labour, but when she took it from her neck and put it against her inner thigh, birth was quick and easy.[32]

Jewish women also used amulets, and this was the case well into the 20th century. In parts of Europe a woman gazed into a bowl of oil, which reflected her face, as in a mirror, and then sent this to the synagogue. The Christian Church was strongly opposed to the use of these amulets. An order was issued in Ireland in County Clare in the 7th century 'that no woman have amber round her neck or have recourse to enchanters . . . or to engravers of amulets'.[33] In their history of childbirth in America, Richard and Dorothy Wertz write that in England practices like these continued for centuries, yet authorities in the Protestant colonies of America eliminated them. 'It seems very likely that the attack on magic undermined and altered women's mysteries and rituals for childbirth. The midwife no longer had a direct charismatic function; she was only to be an effective instrument of God's will. The expectant woman and her attendants could do nothing to seek and offer comfort except to pray to God.'[34]

Throughout the 17th and 18th centuries, devout women who had the education to enable them to keep a journal wrote spiritual testaments as they faced possible death in childbirth, in the same way that men made their will before embarking on a long sea journey or going on a military expedition.[35] Richard and Dorothy Wertz write: 'Women gradually gave to doctors the medical control of birth, the manipulation of their bodies, but they did not give over the rituals of birth. In a compromise that mirrors earlier accommodations between religion and science, women allowed men to treat them as natural machines that might go wrong, but they kept the spiritual meaning of birth for themselves. Social childbirth continued as a divided affair: the body in the hands of men, the spirit in the company of women.'[36]

In most societies birth has been an experience in which, as we shall see in Chapter 4, women draw together to help each other and reinforce bonds in the community. Now that eradication of pain with effective anaesthesia is often the only issue in any discussion of birth – whether to opt for an epidural or go for 'natural' childbirth – the sacramental and social elements which used to be central to women's experience of birth, and still are in some cultures, seem, for an increasing proportion of women, to be completely irrelevant. The journalist Polly Toynbee writes: 'Why the craze for natural childbirth? No-one has started a natural dentistry movement teaching you to meditate

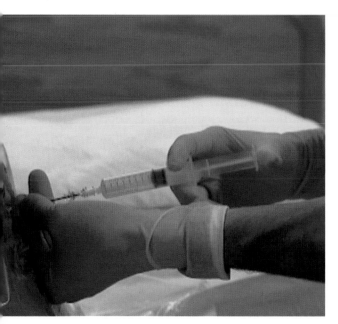

Below: Pain is often the only issue in a discussion of birth – should you opt for an epidural or go for 'natural' childbirth?

through the pain.'[37] One effect of the desanctification of birth is that a woman is left helpless in the face of fear and pain. The guarantee of an epidural as soon as she gets through the hospital door may be the only thing that makes birth bearable.

In every culture birth has been an extraordinary mix of the physiology which is part of our mammalian ancestry – the power of the contracting uterus and beliefs about what it is to be human in relation to the rest of natural creation, the links that bind people together in love and loyalty, and the meaning of life. Birth was segmented from the rest of human experience to become a medical act only in the 20th century, first among the well-to-do and in urban areas in the northern industrial world, and then, as British and American obstetric colonisation spread across the globe, through all social classes, in rural areas and to the rest of the world.

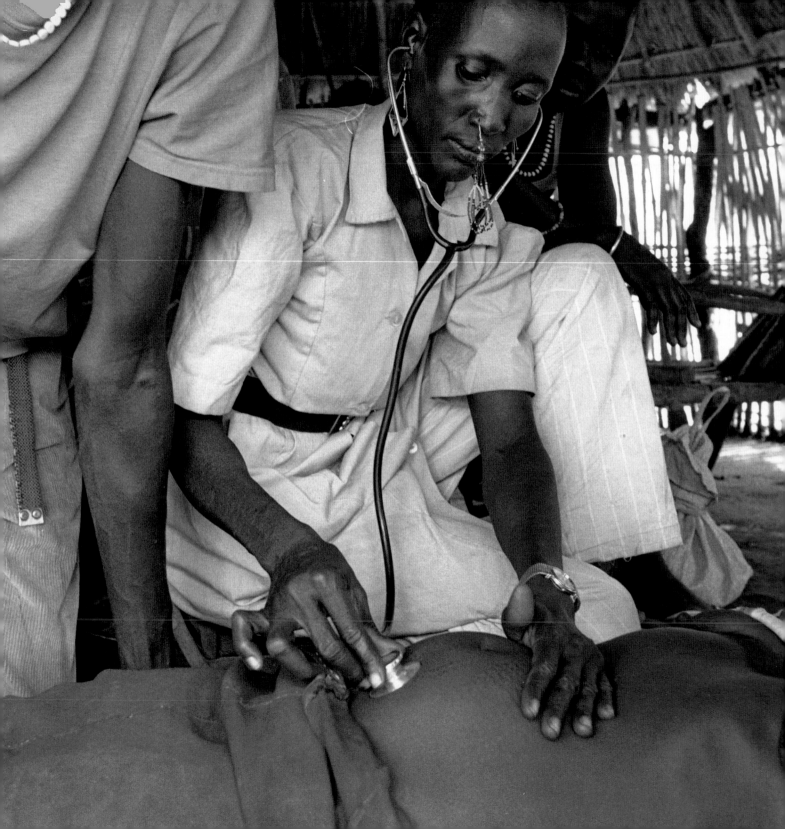

Spiritual Aspects of Birth Today

American granny midwives always looked to the Lord to guide them. A Southern Baptist licensed midwife still practising in the 1990s says, 'I'm from what they call the Bible Belt down there. I'm not ashamed to say that I pray before every birth. Ask the Lord to give us, if it's His will, give us a safe birth and also give me the insight to know in time if I need to ship it out. So I go off to the bathroom – but not for the regular thing [reason] that we go. I go in there and communicate with my Creator. To see if there's something I ought to see.'[38]

In the United States, the virtual death of midwifery in the early 20th century and the take-over by obstetricians has been followed by a revival of midwifery in which midwives must often feel like early Christians in catacombs, resisting a state religion of obstetrics based on a powerful technocracy. Litigation against them not only threatens their livelihood and vocation, but if a baby dies, may land them in prison. The model of birth in hospital is mechanistic. A sociologist, Robbie Pfeufer Kahn, says: 'The social context created by obstetrics denudes childbirth of the sacred.' She believes that most women today lack any language for spiritual experience in birth.[39]

In contrast, midwives interviewed by Penfield Chester, for the most part working outside the hospital system, describe a spiritual way of seeing birth. A midwife from the Oneida nation in Wisconsin says: 'The biggest lesson I learned was the power of spirit . . . As midwives we see that at every delivery. It's just like when God enters you. You shake because the power is so enormous . . . That's usually when the woman says, "I can't do it." Then you know the baby is going to come. As soon as the woman lets go of her control, God comes in, the Power and the Spirit comes in birth. So when I was able to do that with my children – with the second one I did much better – I felt the power of God . . . I think as midwives we're honored with that opportunity to be present when that happens.'[40]

A Muslim midwife says: 'Whenever I go to a delivery, I usually try to take a shower for cleanliness, but also for a Muslim, water has a special meaning, it's called a gushina: you are washing things away from you. And then I make a special prayer before I leave the house that Mosha, the Creator, will show me something that I haven't seen. In the South, when the midwife first came to the house, we all got down on our hands and knees and held hands and prayed. The midwife didn't just go in and take a blood pressure. I like that. I tell people before the birth that I might pray out loud. I pray in Arabic. There is a certain chapter in the Koran that is for complicated births, so I'm working on memorizing that. It's

Left: A traditional birth attendant at work in the Sudan.

important to pray at easy births too. I try to be humble and not attribute success of a birth to myself, but first to God, and then the family, and not get into the ego thing of how I helped you to have your baby. But I'm just there as an aid to the natural process.'[41] A Catholic nun and midwife also says: 'You see miracles happen in your hands and you become faith-filled. You know you didn't do it.'[42] The administrator of the Mennonite Order of the Maternal Services writes: 'I just don't believe that I could do what I do without having a very strong, well-developed religious vein . . . I find myself praying for people, that whatever this mother needs will be there. Praying that guidance will come that will let me know when I need to do something different, like the mother with the ruptured membranes and thick meconium, that kind of stuff. But some wisdom that is higher than my conscious personality would allow me to see that there is a pattern here, and the direction it is leading me is the way to my goal. We constantly have to make choices about what is the right action to take, and how to make those choices I believe to be a religious activity.'[43]

In northern technological cultures today, any spiritual element in childbirth has become a matter of private conviction. Some midwives express religious aspects of their vocation in rather hesitant terms at first: 'I'm not what you would call God-centred, but I believe there is an inner voice. I feel absolutely with the mother but also with the baby. I use this voice – whether it's intuition, I don't know – to guide me.' Yet a Professor of Midwifery, Lesley Page, believes that 'the emergence of new life is a miracle. To me the thing we call God is the power of love, and every baby holds the possibility of knowing and creating love'. For Ina May Gaskin the concept of midwifery is inextricably bound with spirituality. She is the author of the most widely read American midwifery book, *Spiritual Midwifery.*[44]

A midwife who has a sense of the sacred in her work cannot assume that her client shares her values about birth and being. Nor can a mother expect the midwife or doctor to understand what is for her the inner meaning of birth. By lucky chance a midwife and mother may come together who have similar beliefs and a common symbolic language in which to express them. But we have lost the symbols of the spirituality of birth which once linked mother and midwife in a common belief system, and that enabled each birth to be a deeply significant emotional experience for both of them: the rose of Jericho opening its petals in the birth room, the prayers to Mary or to the goddess, symbolic ways of harnessing the power of nature, the ritual untying of knots and opening of doors and windows to help the baby come – all these acts are seen as mere superstition.

In place of them we have our own superstitions about the efficacy of technology, which are as tenacious as any in the Middle Ages. Like the old charms, talismans and invocations, technology is used in the faith that it is bound to make birth safer, whether or not there is any scientific evidence that it achieves that aim. Nine randomised controlled trials have shown that electronic fetal monitoring, for example, does not make birth safer for the baby, compared with intermittent monitoring using a hand-held Doppler or a Pinard's stethoscope (the old midwife's 'trumpet'). Babies are not born in better condition after electronic monitoring, and its use does not reduce the number of babies who need special care. A slightly higher proportion of babies have cerebral palsy when labour is electronically monitored, in fact, and electronic fetal monitoring leads to an increase in Caesarean sections.[45] Yet it is employed in almost every modern hospital all over the world, like a St Christopher medal, to ward off evil and ensure a safe journey.

Northern technological culture has turned birth into a medical event that is conducted in an intensive-care setting. It remains a drama, but it is a hospital drama in which women and their babies are entirely dependent on the life-saving skills of a medical team.

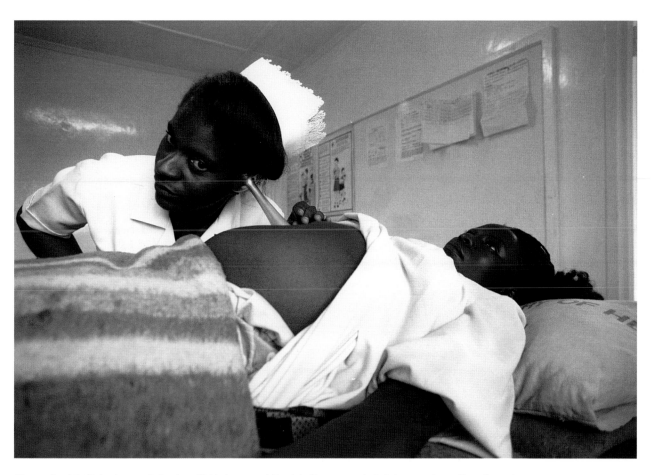

Above: A midwife in the rural district of Ndola, central Zambia, listens to a baby's heart using a Pinard's stethoscope.

Chapter 4

The God-Sibs:
Woman-to-Woman Help

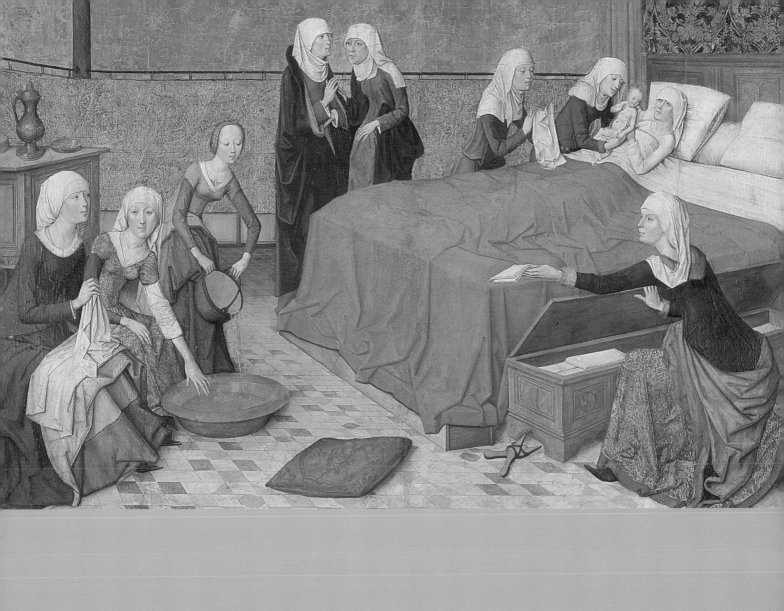

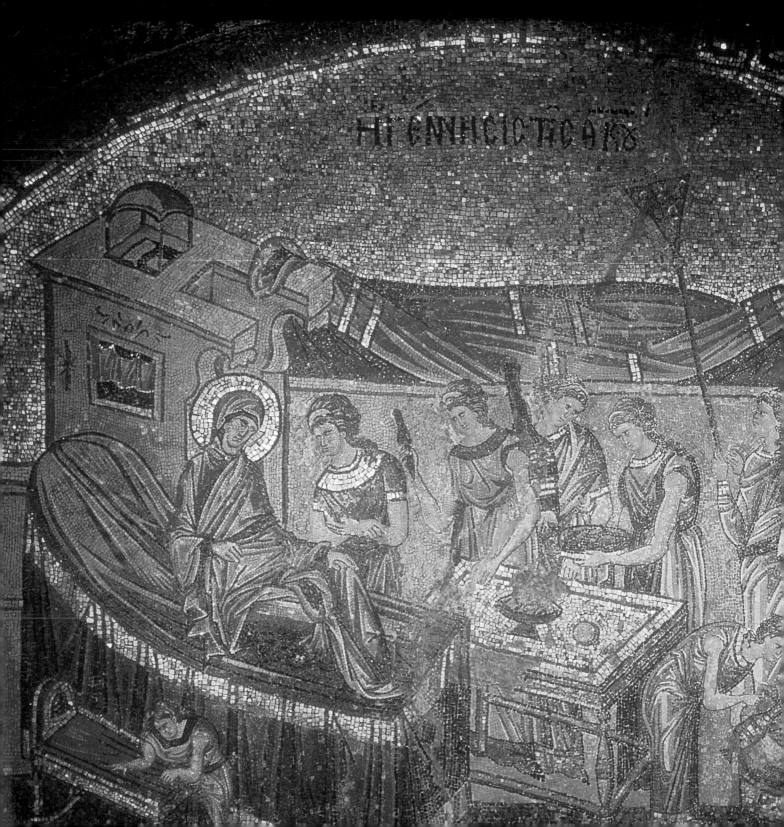

Ἡ ΓΕΝΝΗΣΙΣ ΤΗΣ Θ(ΕΟΤΟ)ΚΟΥ

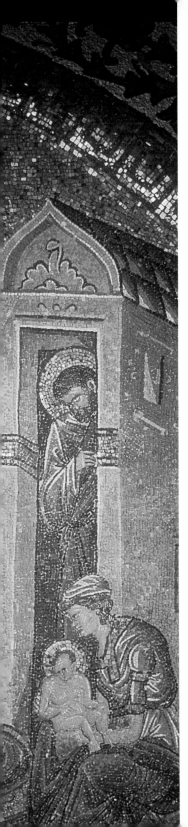

Woman-to-woman help in childbirth is the norm almost everywhere in the world. Men are usually absent, and emotional support, practical help and spiritual succour is offered by women friends, neighbours, in-laws or kin. Social and economic barriers dissolve as women reach out to help each other. It is true that in many rural societies a woman occasionally delivers while on the road to or from market, or while working in the fields, but the normal pattern is for women to draw together.

Exceptions to this are societies in which the ideal birth is one in which a woman goes quietly to a room where she is alone, or into the bush, and comes back with a baby. Michel Odent, the French birth philosopher and surgeon-turned-midwife, believes that solitary birth is the ideal, and is typical of pre-agricultural societies where 'physiological processes were disturbed as little as possible in a human group where the strategy for survival was not to dominate Nature'.[1] In the struggle to control nature 'cultures disturbed the physiological process by denying the mammalian need for privacy'.[2] He describes how companions interfere in labour, disturbing the first contact between mother and baby, and states that 'the greater the social need for aggression and an ability to destroy life, the more intrusive the rituals and beliefs have become in the period surrounding birth'.[3] He cites as an example of a society in harmony with nature the !Kung Sas, an African hunter and gatherer culture, where 'a woman feels the initial stages of labor and makes no comment, leaves the village quietly when birth seems imminent, walks a few hundred yards, finds an area in the shade, clears it, arranges a soft bed of leaves, and gives birth while squatting or lying on her side – on her own'.[4]

The Ju/'hoan women of Botswana and Namibia, in southern Africa, also have such an ideal. But it is important to distinguish between ideal and practice. For it is only with a second birth that a woman is likely to give birth alone; the first time there is a group of women helpers. In this tribe great emphasis is put on independence and personal responsibility and, in striking contrast to the medical model of birth, even when other people help her it is the woman herself who makes the decisions about everything that happens.[5] In West Africa, among the Bariba of the People's Republic of Benin, unassisted, solitary birth is also the ideal. But in practice only 14 per cent of first time mothers deliver alone and 43 per cent of those who already have a child.[6]

Left: A 14th-century Turkish mosaic showing the birth of the Virgin Mary. St Anne is attended by her god-sibs.

After the birth the mother calls another woman to cut the cord. Childbirth is considered a normal and healthy condition, not an illness, but a woman asks others to assist if she is especially afraid, if she had a bad experience last time, or if she had problems.

Marked differences in birth cultures often co-exist even within the same society. In some rural towns of the Peruvian Andes, for example, the baby's father helps during childbirth, physically supporting the mother and giving the baby its first bath. But in other towns not far away, men are excluded, as it is believed that their presence is likely to impede the birth. A group of female helpers, together with the woman's mother, encourage and nurture the labouring woman. After birth there is a traditional period lasting from a few days to several weeks when the new mother is attended by her friends, and other women from the community visit bringing gifts of food and sharing their experiences of birth and motherhood.[7] This is the situation in traditional cultures the world over.

The ways birthing women are cared for can be very different from the quiet, intimate birth scenes that we have come to associate with sensitive, skilled midwifery in birth centres and at home births today. Very large female groups may gather. The result is a noisy bustle of activity, sometimes like a party in full swing, with food, drink, eager sharing of news, laughter and ribald jokes. Anthropologists who have been present at a birth often sound quite shocked by the crowds, the banter and gossip in the birth room.

These women share a serious purpose. The practical work of birth is the central reason for their coming together. Yet childbirth is, above all, an opportunity for asserting female solidarity and reinforcing bonds.

There is another element in this, too: the power of women is expressed in the knowledge and symbolic rites of birth-giving. It transcends all differences and conflicts, draws together everyone in the web of the extended family, and links other families in the community. Birth is a *social occasion*. The labouring woman is at the centre of a birthing circle. An Australian Aboriginal woman expressed this by drawing a spiral symbol and said, 'I am joined. We are part of each other.' She contrasted this symbol of connectedness with a symbol of the disconnectedness she witnessed in 'white' society.

Below: A spiral circle drawn by an Australian Aboriginal woman represented 'connectedness'; she contrasted this with a symbol of the 'disconnectedness' in 'white' society.

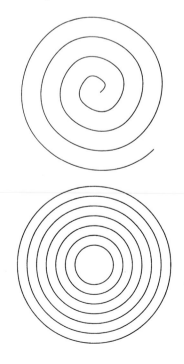

The women work together to help ease the mother's labour, to mark each stage of the journey to life with ritual, and to celebrate the baby's transition to life and the woman's transition to motherhood.

In some cultures only married women attend a birth. In others every female is included, and young girls learn about birth at first hand. An anthropologist who attended a birth in Sarawak said that most of the female members of the village came, including young women who, through watching and helping and sharing in the ritual that followed, learned exactly what happened. She commented: 'Unlike women in the West, few women in this group would give birth not having witnessed and helped with the birth of other babies'.[8]

The women work together to help ease the mother's labour, to mark each stage of the journey to life with ritual, and to celebrate the baby's transition to life and the woman's transition to motherhood. The woman giving birth is the magnetic point that draws them towards her and to each other. Among Bedouin Arabs, for example, the new mother is supposed to stay at home for forty days, and do no cooking or housework, while other women take over her duties. This practice is maintained in urban areas, not only in the countryside. Early in the morning women can be seen leaving their homes, swathed in black cloaks, to visit new mothers and spend half the day drinking tea and coffee and discussing their birth experiences. Each takes a gift of money which she tucks into the newborn's swaddling clothes. When a woman who has visited a mother has *her* next baby, the mother will come to her in return and repay what amounts to a loan. Most of these women are illiterate, but they do very complicated sums to remember who gave exactly what, and work out the interest on it. This is an important way of linking families together, and the anthropologist who described this said that 'women trace out the choreography of the connection between families through their visiting patterns'.[9]

Woman-to-woman help through the rites of passage that are important in every birth has significance not only for the individuals directly involved, but for the whole community. The task in which the women are engaged is *political*. It forms the warp and weft of society.

In Africa and other southern countries where modern clinics provide a medical setting for birth, there is innate conflict between the social and medical versions of birth. The presence of a woman's in-laws or kin is an inconvenience, and may even be considered a danger, so they are often barred from attending. The hospital sets up and guards a medical framework of management.

Abusive Relationships

In North America and Britain domestic violence is common in pregnancy. It is a time when women are least able to defend themselves or take evasive action.[10] In one American study 17 per cent of women had experienced physical or sexual violence, often both, during pregnancy. An abused woman comes to *see* the world and herself through the eyes of her abuser. He is her only reference point in life. There is evidence to show that when a woman has female friends this is far less likely to happen. Having someone in whom to confide and receiving social support from friends protects a woman from violence.

We must not assume that everyone in a traditional culture cares for a woman in pregnancy and childbirth with sensitivity and respect. In a social system in which a bride lives in her husband's parents' household, her in-laws' word may be law. They may treat her like an ignorant child who has no right to make decisions of her own. The women of her husband's family may love and care for her with warmth and gentleness, but, especially if she did not bring a large enough dowry, is suspected of infidelity, or bears daughters rather than sons, they may use their power to deride, punish and abuse her. In acknowledging woman-to-woman help it is important to recognise that power, within the family as elsewhere, can be used vindictively, and that it is not only powerful men who abuse women; women with power may also abuse other women.

In patrilocal marriage, when a woman goes to live with her in-laws, as in large parts of Africa and Asia, the bride is trained in wifely virtues by her mother-in-law. It can be a hard schooling. It is much the same in rural Ireland. In peasant families in the west of Ireland there is an ideal of stoicism in women's lives, and a mother-in-law is often very tough on her son's wife.

There is another kind of violence, too. It is institutional violence. Wherever and with whomever they give birth, women are vulnerable unless information is shared with honesty and they can actively participate in decisions about everything that happens. Any setting in which the providers of care have total control over the management of childbirth can become one in which power is used to abuse women, even though this is done 'for the sake of the baby' or 'for their own good'. Here, too, woman-to-woman support and the information that women share protects against violence. In some cultures a woman knows nothing about birth until she has her baby. But in many, attendance at other women's births in the village means that not only does a woman know what can be done to help, but she is prepared for all the emotional aspects of labour and birth that might otherwise be overwhelming. Understanding of physiological and psychological aspects of the experience of birth is shared by all those participating. This empowers women against violence.

Woman-to-Woman Help in the Past

In different cultures all over the world, women are bonded together in a nurturing act. With the birth of the first baby a woman who was a stranger is no longer a newcomer, but part of a tightly knit family of wives and sisters. The care given to her by the other women during the birth helps forge these bonds.

The helping women, whether the mother's own kin, her in-laws, or neighbours and friends, employ skills that are handed down from mothers to daughters, which link them in both practical and esoteric knowledge denied to men. They share an understanding that is embedded in the female culture which combines spiritual beliefs with empirical knowledge. This knowledge includes prayers, charms, sacred objects and actions which through spiritual agency cause a woman's body to open, such as untying knots and opening windows. Girls learn about these things as soon as they are old enough to help by bringing water, serving food and drink, and doing other chores in the birth room. This is often one of the privileges and responsibilities that come with puberty.

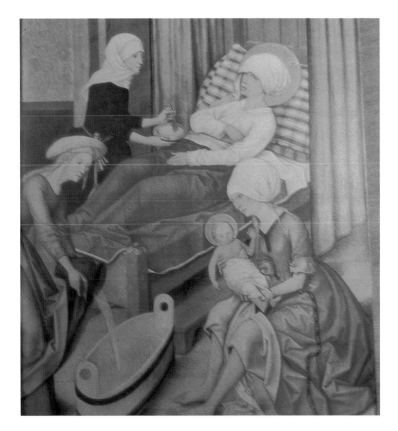

Left: Three helping women care for a mother and baby in this 15th-century painting.

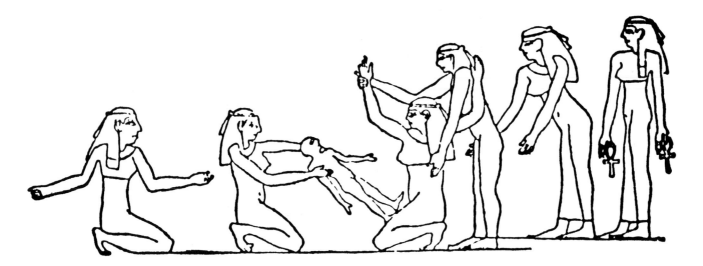

An Egyptian bas-relief shows Cleopatra giving birth with five women assisting. One of them is holding two *ankh*, the keys of life.

Throughout Europe in mediaeval times a woman called on friends and neighbours to attend her in childbirth and care for her in the days afterwards. If need be, some of them stayed for weeks, doing the cooking, washing, looking after the other children, seeing that the necessary tasks in the dairy, herb-garden or smallholding were carried out, and in a peasant household, milking the cow and feeding the pigs and chickens. These women were known as god-sibs – literally 'sisters in God'. Birth took place within female territory, from which men were excluded. They left the house and the women took over. The word god-sib gradually changed in male language to 'gossip'.

Sienese paintings of the 14th century, depicting the births of St John to the aged Elizabeth and of Mary to St Anne, always show these god-sibs nurturing the mother, presenting her with a dish of eggs, chicken or hot broth, the traditional foods for a new mother, and bathing and swaddling the baby. Sometimes there were just two or three women, but often there were more. A 15th-century painting shows three helping women caring for a mother and baby. Much later, German woodcuts show large groups of helping women, one of whom would have been the midwife, bathing and swaddling a new-born baby and supporting the mother.

Above: An ancient Egyptian bas-relief shows Cleopatra giving birth helped by five women.

Right: A woodcut of a Renaissance birth scene with god-sibs. There is a party atmosphere.

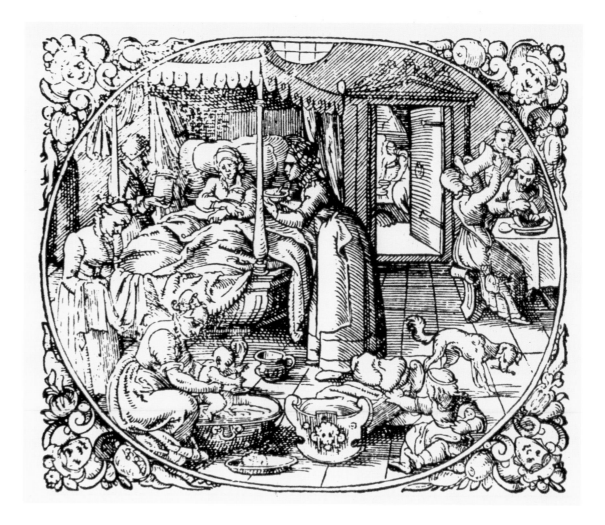

The arrival of god-sibs often heralded an extended party, with much exchange of news, and the jollification might go on for days. In a Renaissance birth scene there is a homely clutter of household items, a dog, an older child with a doll rocking the cradle, women bringing food and what looks like a hot water bottle for the mother, and women at a table, described in the German midwifery text book from which this illustration was taken as 'a jolly company of housewives', who are tucking into a meal and drinking from great flagons.

Social childbirth was the norm in all sections of society. In an illustration of a gypsy birth, the mother is cradled in women's arms, a small child is running to see the baby's head appear, and the father is ready with sustaining food and drink for his wife.

This bustle of female activity, the synchronised rhythms of women in work they know well, is in striking contrast to the isolation which Mary suffered at the birth of Jesus. To the Sienese and Florentine mediaeval mind, it was not just that she gave birth in poverty, but that she was without woman-to-woman support. This was seen as a terrible deprivation. For some mediaeval artists it was inconceivable that Mary should have delivered without help from other women. In a French 15th-century *Book of Hours*, two women are shown, with Joseph watching, looking miserable and bewildered. Joseph looks bemused and quite clearly out of place in Spanish altar paintings of the 13th century, too, in which only the animals are present at the holy birth.

Sometimes the artist depicts a crowd of angels, who in a spiritual sense may have been intended as a substitute for the god-sibs. For it is inconceivable that a woman should be alone in childbirth. Occasionally, midwives are shown hastening to the stable.

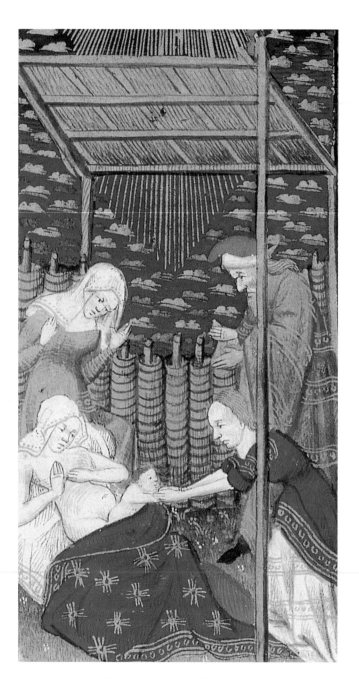

Above: Mary gives birth in the stable with a midwife and another helping woman.
(From a French 15th-century *Book of Hours*.)

Below: 'The birth of Christ' from the Basilica of St Francesco, Rome, with a crowd of angels around the stable.

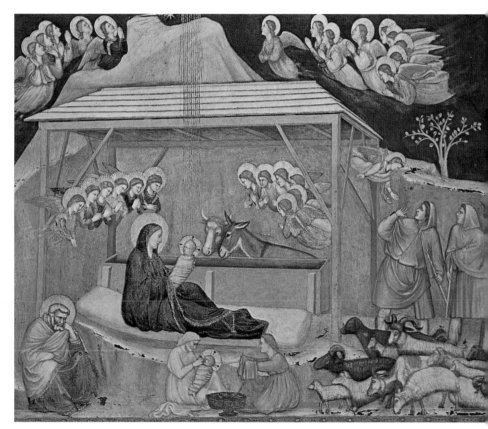

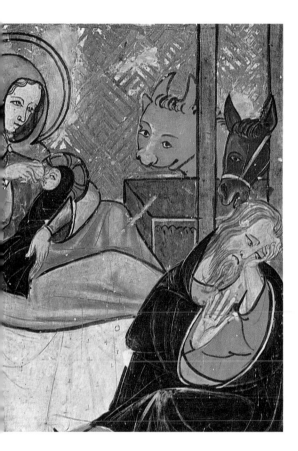

Above: 13th-century Spanish altar painting in which Joseph looks clearly out of place.

The Byzantine tradition is rather different. The story told in the Apocrypha is that when Mary went into labour Joseph left the stable to find help, but when he returned with two midwives she had already delivered. In Byzantine mosaics Mary has two midwives with her. The first midwife examined Mary and said, 'She is a virgin.' The other, Salome, could not believe it and insisted on examining her too. The legend goes that as she withdrew her hand, it withered. An angel appeared and told her to worship the baby and to touch him. The moment she touched the Christ child her hand was healed.[11]

Accounts of woman-to-woman help appear in men's diaries of the Tudor and Stuart period in England: 'Mother Wright the midwife of the parish and . . . nine other honest women attended the birth of George Brown in 1569.'[12] Agnes Bowker was an unwed mother and servant. Yet there were six helping women and the midwife at the birth. Some of these had new babies themselves and came with their babies in their arms. In his diary for 1648 Ralph Josselin writes: 'My wife was delivered of her second son, the midwife not with her, only four women and Mrs Mary.'[13]

In the *Batchelars Banquets*, a translation of a French work, there is a satire on childbirth. The man is no longer master in his own home and complains, 'When the time draws near of her lying down, then must he trudge to bid gossips, such as she will appoint, or else all the fat is in the fire.' His house is over-run by chattering 'sisters, wives, aunts, cousins' and other women feasting, carousing and running down all his household resources. They return for the ceremonies of upsitting (when the mother gets out of bed) and churching. It is a costly affair.[14]

Some Tudor town councils tried in vain to control the activities of gossips. Chester city ruled against gossips completely 'for as much as great excess and superfluous costs and charges hath and doth daily grow by reason of costly dishes, meats and drinks brought unto women lying in childbed'.[15] A Jacobean preacher published a book of devotions which included a prayer that those attending a woman in childbirth 'avoid at this time effeminate speeches, wanton behaviour, and unseasonable mirth, which often doth accompany such meetings as this'.[16]

Throughout history, until well into the middle of the 20th century in many countries, birth was women's work, and every woman has been expected to know what to do. Helping in childbirth was an extension of the skills of mothering and involved the arts of healing that were required of an adult woman. Each had her herbs and 'simples', and special teas to soothe or stimulate, to heat or to cool the blood. Only the aristocracy or the wealthiest tradespeople turned to male midwives and to the barber surgeons who had the right to use instruments to deliver, or to dismember, a baby. Usually, even though a man might be present at birth, he was marginal. He might be a male astrologer to foretell the child's future from the position of the stars at the moment of birth. But women did the practical birthing work.

Helping in childbirth was an extension of the skills of mothering.

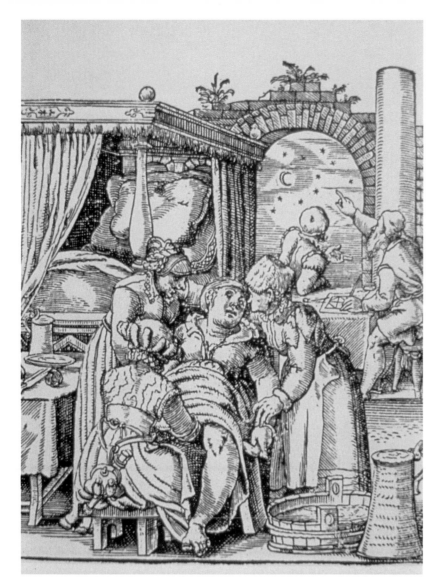

Left: A woodcut. Two men are present, but their function is to record the position of the stars at the moment of birth. The women get on with the work.

North America

The social nature of birth was reinforced with the colonisation of North America. But as people emigrated from a Europe in turmoil to seek new lands, journeying in pioneer wagons and building log cabins, North American women felt keenly the isolation from their female kin. Whenever possible they travelled, sometimes for great distances.

Women on neighbouring farms came together to help each other. Each knew that when they had their next baby, they in turn would be assisted by their neighbours. It was called 'turnabout' help. They gathered to sew bed quilts and baby clothes and took over the work in the house and the barn after the birth until the mother was up and about. At the end of pregnancy a woman had to stock up with food and drink to prepare for entertaining what was often a large group of women. One woman said that you never knew how long they would stay and you couldn't pay these friends, so you had to make sure to treat them well.

A man wrote in his diary that seventeen women attended his wife.[17] Ebenezer Parkman similarly recorded that six women came to help when his wife was 'brought to bed' in 1738.[18] This was often incredibly difficult for women to achieve. Their families were spread geographically far apart, swift transport did not yet exist, and in rural areas the nearest neighbours might be miles away. They overcame overwhelming obstacles in order to be with each other. Judith Leavitt, an authority on birth in America in the 18th and 19th centuries, comments:

Except the most desperate poor who were forced by circumstances into institutions for their confinements, all American birthing women had access to this network to varying degrees, depending on their locale and their own social acquaintances. Women often went to help other women whom they hardly knew; when the call for help came, women responded. The women's support network that was activated when a pregnant woman found herself ready to deliver her child was impressive; and it was renewed each time a woman in the neighborhood went into labor.[19]

In the 17th and 18th centuries in New England, the first stage of labour was rather like a party, and women arrived with gifts of groaning cakes and groaning beer to add to the mother's store. It was the custom to throw a groaning party at the end of the lying-in, too. One woman served 'Boil'd Pork, Beef, Fowls: very Good Rost Beef, Turkey Pye, Tarts' to seventeen women who had attended her.[20]

A pregnant woman usually wanted her mother with her most of all. But that was often impossible. Women wrote to their mothers who remained in Europe or on the East Coast, looking for support at least through letters. 'If you could be with me now, what wouldn't I give . . . '; 'Dearest Mother mine. All would be complete if you were here.'[21] Sometimes women travelled enormous distances to be with their mothers. They might ride fifty miles or more and return on horseback with the new baby. Dorothy Lawson McCall went from Oregon to Massachusetts and back with every one of her four births.[22]

Only if a woman could not find support from other women did she turn to her husband for help. Though men and women's lives intertwined, they were in many ways separate. Men knew nothing of childbirth, menstruation, breastfeeding, pregnancy, menopause and 'women's troubles'. Women's fears and hopes might be discussed by close friends and family members when they got together, but men did not share this female knowledge. It was as if men and women lived in different worlds.

Yet with the colonisation of new lands, the fanning out of a population as pioneers crossed the continent and young families moved through vast tracts of land to establish new settlements, and with the search for economic prosperity in distant towns, from New England to California and from the Deep South to the Canadian border, that had to change. Men started to be involved in women's lives in a new way. They often did this reluctantly, and only in emergencies, but it was a fundamental switch in the relationship between a man and woman.

In 1908 a logger's wife described her breech birth:

When Bill was gone once . . . I broke water and was having too much pain. Feeling that baby with my hands I knew for certain it was going to be breech. I put the kids to bed to keep warm and told the older ones keep that fire going no matter what . . . I got on a pallet under my quilts and Lordy did I pray for Bill to come back. He came blowing in that night. He pulled that baby out.[23]

Doctors

When women were socially isolated like this, without female friends, and there was no midwife, the way was open for doctors to take over childbirth. As immigrants established themselves on the new continent, built successful farming enterprises and businesses, and prospered economically, the demand for doctors grew. From the 1760s on, the colonists started to turn from midwives, who represented the old European ways of birthing, to male doctors. It was a sign of social status to be able to afford a doctor. Medical men had high prestige and a man was automatically assumed to be better educated than any woman, whether or not he had been to medical school (and most practising doctors had not), and whether or not he had learned anything about childbirth in medical school (which was also doubtful). The doctors were general practitioners. The practice of obstetrics was attractive to aspiring doctors, because once they had safely delivered a baby there was the opportunity of becoming the family physician. Obstetrics set doctors up for building a practice.

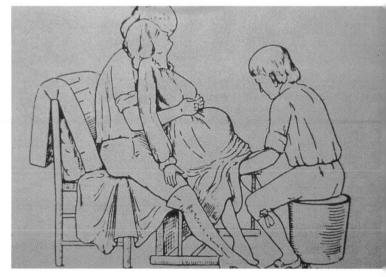

Above: Colonial America. A doctor is delivering the baby and the woman is supported between her husband's thighs.

Even when a doctor attended, it was expected that there would be at least one other woman present to assist. In New England she helped to prepare the *borning room*. This was a special small room behind the stove, warm and secluded, that was kept for births.

Women actively negotiated what they wanted with the doctor, and the ideas of other women in the family, as well as those of friends and neighbours who were present, were all considered. A doctor in Oklahoma wrote to the journal of the American Medical Association in 1912 saying that it was impossible to shave women's pubic hair because these women objected to the practice.

In about three seconds after the doctor has made the first rake with his safety (razor), he will find himself on his back out in the yard with the imprint of a woman's bare foot emblazoned on his manly chest, the window sash around his neck and a revolving vision of all the stars in the firmament [sic] presented to him.

  'Tell him not to try to shave m'.'[24]

Another doctor in Kansas regretted that it was impossible to get sterile conditions in the home because of the presence of five or six neighbours and, perhaps, the mother of the patient. Doctors complained that nothing could be done without the women's consent and urged that everyone but the patient should be turned out of the birth room. A doctor's social prestige depended largely on the opinion that these friends and neighbours formed of him. If there was only one doctor in the area, a woman obviously had little or no choice, though it is recorded that one woman in California was delighted to have the doctor's wife with her, but absolutely refused to allow the doctor through the door.

It was taken for granted that women in labour were upright, moved around, and used rafters, ropes, window ledges and furniture to get into comfortable positions. A husband could help with this, and a woman might give birth sitting between his thighs.

A major cause of maternal death after childbirth was infection, and doctors added to this risk. When women assisted at birth they relied on encouragement and emotional support, helping the mother change position and move about, applying hot and cold compresses, and giving herbal medications and massage. They did not put their hands inside to try and turn the baby's head and they used no instruments to expedite delivery. Some doctors prided themselves on applying forceps before full dilatation of the cervix because they claimed it saved the mother nervous exhaustion and pain.

The more a doctor busied himself with birth interventions the greater the chance of infection. In the USA birth became increasingly dangerous at the beginning of the 20th century, by which time doctors were delivering around half of all babies, and this remained the case until the discovery of antibiotics in the 1930s. Many maternal deaths attributed to tuberculosis were in fact due to childbirth sepsis.

In the absence of other women, and with only a single care-giver, women were confined to bed during childbirth because that was the easiest place for a doctor to keep an eye on them, and they could maintain their modesty by being covered in bedding. The male take-over of childbirth posed a dilemma concerning modesty. It has been described as 'a social event that challenged codes of purity and privacy' and 'an initiation rite . . . a moral test and a physical trial in which the male doctor . . . judged a woman's passage into adult society'.[25]

England

In England during the same historical period, the vast majority of mothers were cared for by midwives, many of whom were highly skilled, although most women also continued to have the help of neighbours, family and friends in both urban and rural areas. Knowledge about childbirth was transmitted orally and could not be found in books. The only written advice about what to do was from men, who usually learned what they could from midwives, passed on fragments from medical texts dating from antiquity, and some of whom had had the opportunity to dissect a female corpse in medical school. Men's diaries and medical books make it clear that childbirth drew women together to help the mother. A book called *Medical Knowledge*, which is undated but appears to be a late 18th- or early 19th-century edition of a much earlier publication, refers to 'the good women' who gave the mother physical support and assisted her in moving around rather than lying in bed. Long before the term 'active childbirth' was coined, these women helped the labouring woman stay upright and mobile. She should 'walk about her chamber as much as she can, the women supporting her under the arms, if it be necessary; for by this means the weight of the child causeth the inward orifice of the womb to dilate the sooner than in bed; and if her pains be stronger and more frequent, labour will not be near so long'.[26]

Birth started to be medicalised in the late 19th century. In England, as in the USA, medicalised birth was more dangerous than social childbirth. Obstetrics was a branch of general practice. Delivering babies 'established a professional man's reputation . . . Deliver the babies and you will have the family as patients for the rest of your life'.[27] There was a great deal of interference, and doctors used chloroform and forceps routinely in otherwise normal labours. As many as 70 per cent of women cared for at home by general practitioners were delivered in this way. In the 1930s, GPs were still applying forceps in 50 per cent or more of births.[28] This made birth very dangerous. Mortality rates in general had started to drop in the late 19th century. But maternal mortality remained at a high level – 500–600 deaths per 100,000 births. Infant mortality had dropped dramatically, but the risk of a woman dying in childbirth was as high in the 1930s as in the mid-19th century.[29]

In every society mortality rates are highest among the poor. The extraordinary thing was that, at that time, in contrast to mortality rates as a whole, the risk of death in childbirth was greatest in the upper and middle classes and lowest in the labouring classes. The well-to-do, who could afford a doctor, were most at risk. At least a third of all maternal deaths were due to bad obstetric practice.[30] As late as 1934, a woman who lived in the area of Kensington, London, and who was delivered by a doctor, was twice as likely to die as a woman in the poorest area, the East End, who was attended by a midwife and had a strong female social support network.

Unnecessary obstetric intervention, combined with streptococcal infection, was a factor in wide international differences in mortality rates. The lowest death rates were in Scandinavia and the Netherlands, the highest in the USA, a country where midwives were despised and doctors delivered most babies. Maternity mortality rates in Britain were halfway between these extremes.

Whenever women gave birth with midwives, woman-to-woman care was central to the experience. A study of midwife-conducted home births in Nottingham in the twenty-four years from the start of the National Health Service in 1948 until its reorganisation in 1982, reveals that 95 per cent of women who delivered at home were cared for entirely by midwives, never visited a hospital and never saw an obstetrician. They received total care from a district midwife, together with practical help and emotional support from neighbours, family and friends.[31] That was vital. The midwife was not a solo performer. She depended on other women to give their assistance, and they worked as a group.

The women who helped at birth were well-versed in the preparation. A large pile of newspapers were collected, some to be put into the bed and others to scatter over the floor while the mother was pacing about in labour in case she should bleed or her membranes rupture over the linoleum or the midwife spill lotion on the floor. Cotton sheets were passed from house to house to use at the delivery and then boiled for the next confinement: old sheets were torn into strips to be used as drawer sheets and some hemmed as cot sheets . . . Supporters knew how to make the delivery bed: a rubber sheet went on the mattress, a boiled cotton sheet went on top, followed by thick layers of newspaper or brown paper between folds of torn sheet, on top of which a drawer sheet would be placed.[32]

What most women achieved from a home birth was to be confined in a loving environment with people of their choice present . . . The mother remained as the head of the household . . . If the midwife's time was scarce, there was always someone to bath the baby and make the bed, but it was the person the woman had chosen who performed the tasks she asked them to do.[33]

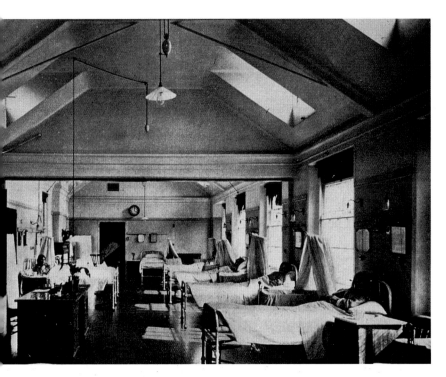

Above: The maternity ward of the Royal Free Hospital, London; c. 1912.

In hospital births during the same period it was unusual for any woman to have a female relation or friend with her; with the move from home to hospital there was no place for it. In the first quarter of the 20th century, midwifery organisations were created and legislation progressively squeezed unlicensed midwives out of practice. Care became more professionalised and women increasingly gave birth in hospital. Female family members, friends and neighbours were seen as intruders in a medical event that had nothing to do with them. Not only were other women excluded from the birth, but doctors claimed that they had a detrimental effect on the pregnant woman's mind.

They were said to spread 'old wives' tales'. In a popular book published in 1975, an obstetrician wrote that everything women said about birth was 'a cartload of rubbish' and warned his readers not to listen 'to wicked women with their malicious, lying tongues'.[34]

Godmothers in Sicily

Female support has been given recognition in Christian culture through godmothers. These are the god-sibs by another name. In the past they attended the birth and accepted spiritual responsibility for the child. It was common for the baby to have a group of godmothers, not just one.

In Sicilian villages the role of the *comare* is still important. I learned about them from Sicilian midwives and doctors who described to me birth practices in Lentino, a village south of Catania, ten miles from the coast, in the province of Syracuse. In Sicilian towns today there is only one godmother for a child. But in rural areas like this several *comare* are selected by the mother from among her neighbours and they attend the birth to support her and to care for the baby. A woman cannot refuse. It is an honour and a social responsibility.

The midwife first hands the baby not to the mother, but to the senior *comare* – an older woman who is a friend of one of the grandmothers. As the baby is born the mother points to her so that it is clear who she is. She wears a special apron, usually white, called the *foura*, in which she cradles the baby. She examines and bathes it and then swaddles it from the feet up in white gauze, with the intention of strengthening the legs and straightening the body. The outer swaddling bands are often lavishly embroidered. She is known as the godmother of the *foura*. The other women present include the *comare* of the booties, the *comare* of the bonnet, and the *comare* of the shirt, who dress the baby in these garments and are responsible for washing them while the woman is lying-in – several days for a peasant mother, eight days for an aristocratic mother. They prepare special dishes for her during this time, chicken or pigeon broth to promote lactation, and toast. The father of the baby has to eat the head and neck of the chicken to help the baby's neck grow straight. Through their attendance at the birth and their assistance afterward, these women have a relationship with the child that lasts through life. They have become 'family'.

The traditional custom is to delay the first breastfeed for twelve hours, during which time the *comare* give prelacteal feeds from a *pipitui*, a muslin dummy that is soaked in sugared water, or dipped in a jelly of *chicoria* to which olive oil, lemon and salt are added.

In many cultures colostrum is seen as too 'strong', or as dangerous, for the newborn. So it is expressed and thrown away, while the baby is breastfed by other women or fed substitute fluids until there is evidence of mature milk. This custom strengthens relationships between women and through them other families in the community. It actively engages other women in the care of mother and baby. The infant is not simply the child of this mother, but of a group of women linked in commitment to each other. This practice denies babies the undoubted benefits of colostrum, but has a cohesive function which is very important, especially in a society in which disease, malnutrition or accident may cut short a mother's life.

Egypt

In Egypt today, the group helping the birthing woman include her mother, her husband's mother, her husband's sisters, her own sisters, paternal aunts and perhaps a neighbour as well as the midwife. They hold her in their arms or support her back in a squatting, kneeling or sitting position, depending on how she is most comfortable at the time and what the midwife advises.

They also make sure that she has food. Eggs are believed to increase the body's heat, which is what the woman in labour needs, and they also feed her egg after the birth; one woman cradles her while another places the food in her mouth. In labour they concentrate entirely on the birthing mother during each contraction and give words of encouragement. Between contractions they chat about their own childbirth experiences and the tasks of planting and harvesting. They coax her to go on and have courage when her morale drops, taking turns to hug and kiss her and say, 'Be strong my love'; 'I wish it was I giving birth'; 'Just a little longer and it will be over my love'; 'Be brave sweet one, finish, you are almost there sweet one.'[35]

After the baby is born they wash the mother and tie her hair in a kerchief. They care for the child, rejoicing if it is a boy and sharing the mother's disappointment if it is a girl. It is believed that 'a woman's grave is open until the fortieth day', and a new mother must have rest and high protein food during this time, when both mother and baby are at risk of the Evil Eye. So the women who attended the birth also look after mother and baby in the weeks following. Or at least, this is the ideal. In practice, only the wealthiest women can avoid housework and work in the fields for this long.

Mexico

The Seri are a small tribe who live in one of the driest, poorest areas of Mexico. Most women are now transported to hospital to have their babies, but there is a strong tradition of woman-to-woman help.

The Seri mother decides who she wants with her at the birth. Occasionally this is just one helper, but an anthropologist attending a birth commented, with some surprise, 'I counted sixteen women and children, most of whom were sitting around in an aura of fiesta.'[36] The usual practice is to have at least two women: 'she who raises her up', who kneels on the ground with her legs spread wide apart so that the birthing woman can sit in her lap, leaning backward, resting her head on her shoulder, and 'one who grabs up', who holds her hand on the ground beneath the skirt of the labouring woman, to catch the baby when it is born. They are usually close relatives. There are other women ready to take their place if birth is long and tiring, and women waiting to massage the mother immediately after the baby is born and before the placenta is delivered. The helper who 'raises her up' changes position with the mother's movements, and occasionally both women will help her stand if she wishes to.

They prepare special teas to help the birth, and after the baby is delivered they bind a long piece of cloth tightly around the mother's fundus to aid the expulsion of the placenta, massage her abdomen, and give her other special teas. Once the placenta is delivered they wrap hot stones in cloth or heat bundles of twigs and place them against her body to ease after-pains. The baby is washed and dressed and one of the women offers sweetened water from a clam shell and rests the baby in the mother's arms. They also have the task of keeping a ritual fire burning in the home for four days after the birth in order to 'fire' the baby, much as a clay pot is fired in a kiln. Since neither parent is supposed to work for at least four days after the birth, these women take on the household tasks, though in practice the father usually has to get back to the fields and the mother does a little light washing. But it is the women helpers who keep the home running.

The Inuit

Today most Inuit women in northern Canada are not allowed to give birth in their own communities. They are transported to a large regional hospital many hundreds of miles away, in Winnipeg, for example, where they have to deliver their babies among total strangers. They are evacuated to the city some time toward the end of pregnancy and must spend the intervening period away from their families in a lodging house.

Previously they gave birth with the help of their mothers and mothers-in-law, together with other female family members and neighbours, and often their husbands as well. There were usually at least three helping women present and the father was much more actively involved in the birth than is the case today. Before they lived in settlements women gave birth in igloos, tents and temporary log cabins, sometimes in the open, in boats and even on moving sledges. Knowledge about birth was shared among all those who helped and in many camps there was no particular individual with specialised training. Every woman was educated to assist.

A woman from Whale Cove said that her mother taught her to come to the aid of any woman who was in labour 'because it can happen at any time and you might be alone with your family . . . when there are no other women around'.[37] Learning how to help at birth was part of the preparation for womanhood. From childhood on, girls were told exactly what happened and were present when their mothers and other women gave birth. Another explained, 'We did not need to be taught what to do; we did things as we had seen done'.[38]

One woman described a birth in which three men were commanded to leave because they were thought to be blocking the child's exit. It was considered important that a woman could be relaxed and comfortable with whoever was present during her labour and she was free to ask anyone to go away.[39]

Attempts are being made to rediscover birth traditions and to train Inuit midwives. The Pauktuutit, the Inuit Women's Association of Canada, has resolved to establish birthing facilities in all Inuit communities so that women can give birth without having to leave their families.

> **It was considered important that a woman could be relaxed and comfortable with whoever was present during her labour and she was free to ask anyone to go away.**

Japan

Japan has a strong tradition of woman-to-woman help in childbirth. Beside the midwife, the *samba*, both grandmothers often assisted, together with other women from the neighbourhood. Still today, a woman may go to her mother's house a month before the birth and, although she usually has a hospital delivery, is cared for by her mother and female relatives. But in the big cities, such as Osaka, less than 10 per cent now return to their mother's homes. It remains an ideal, but one that is difficult to put into practice.[40]

In their own homes women are supposed to work hard and serve the needs of their husband and children. Pregnant women are advised to engage in hard, physical work to make birth easier. As a result, it is difficult for a pregnant woman who does not go home to her mother to have any rest. If she can afford it she may check into a 'love hotel' that lets rooms at an hourly rate, simply for an afternoon's rest. Up to 50 per cent of the clientele of these 'love hotels' consists not of men wanting quick sex, but of housewives desperate for a chance to sleep.

Most historical records describe birth in noble households, so peasant birth may have been rather different, but all accounts make it clear that woman-to-woman help was central to birth. Surviving descriptions of peasant birth suggest that the pregnant woman built her own birth hut, went into it when labour started, and lived there for some weeks afterwards. During this time she was free of household chores and was cared for by other women. When she was in active labour all the married women of the village gathered and shouted and grunted with her. This was called *goriki* (sharing). After the birth there was a celebratory meal. Rice was cooked, and once it had been offered to the God of Birth, was fed to the mother and then distributed by the midwife to those who had helped.

Accounts from the Heian era (794–1192) tell how the women used to spread a bear-skin on the floor of the birth hut (because bears give birth with ease), sprinkle it with ashes, and place a *titani* mat and sheets over it so that the woman could deliver on them. From the earliest historical time and through the Middle Ages, all the women helpers wore white, a lucky colour. When a woman was in labour they plucked bow strings to make a buzzing sound to drive evil away. As she started to push one woman supported her pelvis and another threw rice, a fertility symbol, into the air to help the birth. If there were difficulties a woman smashed open earthen vessels or cedarwood boxes to help the labouring woman's body open. After the birth it was one woman's task to massage the newborn baby.

Today, most women have their babies in large hospitals, but there are a growing number of small clinics run and staffed by midwives, and slightly larger clinics run by women obstetricians and staffed by midwives, which have recreated an all-female environment for birth. Birth in the midwife-run clinics are called 'home births' because they are based in the midwife's own home. There are one or two rooms with *titani* mats on the floor and a delivery chair. Little intervention of any kind takes place. No drugs are used, no episiotomies performed, and the father is welcome. After the birth the midwife places futons on the floor so that the parents can sleep with their baby. One mother told me, 'She didn't take the baby away unless you wanted. She said, "When you feel like going home you can go home." They did whatever I said.'

Toho Women's Clinic in Tokyo is run by a woman obstetrician. The birth room here also has mats on the floor, a futon and a birth stool. Nearby there is a room with a birth chair. The obstetrician tells me that in the year preceding our meeting there were no forceps or vacuum extractions and only three out of twenty women had a small episiotomy. Though she rarely does inductions, she sometimes stimulates the cervix with laminaria pods. These have seeds that swell when they absorb water, and are traditionally used to help dilatation if the woman is very slow in labour.

In these clinics, in each of which there are not more than around 200 births a year, there is a strong sense of female companionship and co-operation. They represent a contrast to the ethos and management style of the big hospitals where the obstetrician is 'master', *sensei*, and the midwife is addressed as 'the obstetrician's assistant', *josanpu*, rather than *sanba-san*, the term used by independent midwives and those who work outside the hospitals.

The Netherlands

Dutch birth culture has always been woman-centred, but has usually involved the father of the baby as well. In the 17th century the Netherlands developed a unique culture of domesticity in comfortable, prosperous merchant homes in the towns. There was nothing like it anywhere else in Europe. The conjugal family, with its emphasis on individual relationships in a setting of intimacy, became the basic social unit. Visitors from other countries marvelled at the cleanliness, order and serenity of Dutch homes. Until then little value was set on privacy, households were large, and important decisions were made in the community rather than in the nuclear family.

This change is expressed in the many paintings of homely domestic scenes which we know as 'the Dutch school'. One genre of painting very popular among private collectors was the peaceful birth room or *kraamkamer* scene. Women friends and family members were usually present to help the mother and baby. The huge groups of women characteristic of birth scenes in the early 17th century in the Netherlands, and later in Italy and Germany, were absent. And the father is often present not just as an onlooker, but as an integral member of the group. Late 17th- and 18th-century *kraamkamer* paintings depict the intimate circle around the mother and baby.[41]

For many Dutch women birth remains a domestic process and they go through the whole of their pregnancy and birth without seeing a doctor. Thirty per cent of births still take place at home. The state

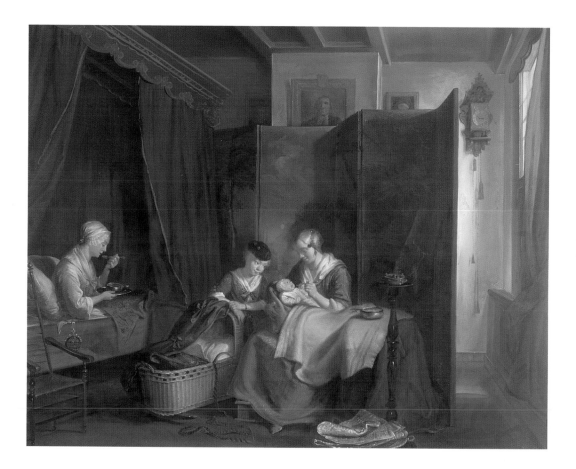

Left: A *kraamkamer* painting. 'The Nursery' by Cornelius Troost, 1737.

also provides women helpers who come into the home, supplementing or taking the place of the care given by female family members. This training was first established at the turn of the century, because with rapid urbanisation couples often moved to towns where they had no other family. In 1926 the government started to sponsor the scheme nationally and it remains an important part of maternity care. The helping woman, or *kraamverzorgende*, assists during the birth, cares for the mother and baby afterwards, and does the housekeeping and cooking. An American sociologist, Barbara Katz Rothman, describes her meeting with one of these women:

The door was opened by someone I took to be the baby's aunt. She was washing up from lunch and was about to pick up the older child from a friend's house. She told us the mother, father and baby were sleeping upstairs. Only later did I learn that she was the maternity aide – but this was not help one buys if rich or borrows from friends and family if not, but the birthright of all Dutch families.[42]

The Rediscovery of Woman-to-Woman Care

There is developing awareness in modern hospitals of the value of woman-to-woman support through labour. It is not only that mothers are happier when they have another woman with them; birth is easier and safer. Female companionship is the one element in care which has been shown to be most effective in keeping birth normal. The term often used is doula, first suggested by the anthropologist Dana Raphael.[43]

No other interventions that have been introduced and experimented with over the last thirty years have had such success in systematically reducing the rate of Caesarean sections and leading to better outcomes for mother and baby. Eleven randomised controlled trials, most of them in hospitals where women normally have little or no emotional support, reveal that companionship by another woman during labour results in mothers needing fewer pain-relieving drugs and having fewer instrumental deliveries and Caesarean sections. Babies are in better condition at birth, too.[44]

The first study took place in Guatemala, in a large hospital where there was an enormous gulf between the impersonal way in which patients were usually treated and the care they would have had from women family members and friends and the local midwife in their villages.[45] This was followed by research in the United States by the same team. It was carried out in a busy, high-tech hospital in Houston, Texas, that caters for Hispanic, black and white women, all of them of low income and without insurance. They are usually not allowed to have any support person with them during childbirth, though family members may get permission to pop in and out. Patients are confined to bed and have continuous electronic fetal monitoring (EFT), intravenous infusions, artificial rupture of the membranes, frequent oxytocin stimulation of the uterus, and epidurals and other forms of pharmacological pain relief – the standard menu of American hospital care of women who are poor and from ethnic minorities.

The women who gave support had all experienced normal births themselves, received a three-week training, and stayed with the mother from admission until after the birth. They were not present as representatives of the hospital, but simply as friends. They explained to the mother what was happening physiologically, and soothed, touched and encouraged her. This companionship had the effect of reducing rates of complications and interventions. The supported women had less augmentation of labour, fewer epidurals, more spontaneous deliveries and fewer Caesareans, and their babies had a shorter hospital stay. The researchers concluded that support of this kind is a simple, cost-effective way of enhancing well-being for mothers and babies.[46]

All the research into women's feelings about companionship reveals that they find labour better than they expected and think back to the birth as a positive experience.[47;48] Some studies show that women are less likely to have perineal tears or episiotomies.[49] They are also more likely to be breastfeeding exclusively when the baby is six weeks old, even though in South Africa, where this particular research took place, the labour companions did not visit the postnatal ward and never discussed breastfeeding with the mothers. What seems to have happened is that women's self-confidence increased and this enabled them to breastfeed successfully.[50] That is not all. Women are also less likely to be depressed six weeks after birth[51], and face fewer emotional problems with mothering.[52]

The latest research has been done in Botswana, where women have always gone back to their mothers' homes to give birth, but where nowadays, when they give birth in hospitals, relatives are not allowed to be present. A randomised controlled trial there revealed that having a birth companion reduced the rate of all obstetric interventions, including Caesarean sections.[53]

Each one of these studies has examined the effects of woman-to-woman companionship – not support by a male partner. While there is research which shows that a male partner's presence reduces the need for pain-relieving drugs, few randomised controlled trials have examined male participation. No studies have reported any decrease in rates of augmentation of labour or of forceps deliveries or Caesarean sections when male partners were present. John Kennell and Marshall Klaus suggest that it may be difficult for a man to give adequate emotional support when he is deeply emotionally involved himself and lacks direct personal experience of birth.

American research comparing the kind of support given by first-time fathers and by doulas, revealed that women touch the mother 95 per cent of the time, but men only 20 per cent of the time that they are present, and also that men choose to be there for shorter periods.[54] Whether or not this is true for all men – and it is unwise to generalise across cultures – Klaus and Kennell consider that a father should not have to be the sole support person in the birth room: 'The presence of additional support in the form of an experienced woman, far from diminishing the role of the father, can enhance it by reducing his anxiety and freeing him to offer more personal support.'[55]

The Father's Role

In cultures in which birth takes place in the world of women and from which the father is excluded, he may either have a clearly defined and important role or be left stranded and anxious. He goes off to the pub with his mates to drink the time away, and after a phone call to the hospital that tells him he is now a father he 'wets the baby's head' with yet more alcohol. Or he sits in the fathers' waiting room, staring at the TV and smoking to try to calm his nerves. If there are other children, perhaps he lends a hand with them, often under the direction of his mother-in-law who has come to stay.

In Britain, since the 1960s, approximately ten years earlier than in the United States, fathers have been welcome in delivery rooms. This has not always worked to the woman's advantage. While midwives and

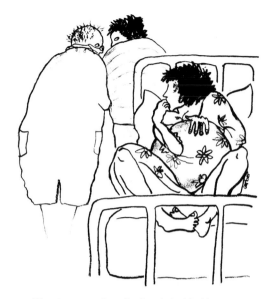

'The doctor and my husband decided between them that I should have an epidural.'

doctors readily accepted fathers, male doctors sometimes formed a liaison with a man which, in effect, excluded the woman from making her own decisions about what she wanted. The men made decisions for her and sometimes managed the birth together in an aura of male camaraderie.

Although one father handcuffed himself to a Chicago delivery table to stay with his wife for the birth of their baby, throughout the 1960s and 1970s in the United States the father was likely to be turned out of the delivery room when the woman started to push.

Meanwhile, in Britain the presence of the baby's father was so much accepted that some men felt under pressure to be there when they did not want to. Hospital staff were adept at incorporating fathers into the birth scene. The real bugbear of many hospital staff was not the male partner, but the woman's mother. Through this period it was more difficult for female family members to get permission to attend a birth. In discussions with midwives, concern was expressed about the harm that a mother could do with her old-fashioned ideas and her uncontrolled fear if she attended her daughter's birth.[56] In fact, many men felt alien in delivery rooms, bewildered by hospital practices, and because of their anxiety were unable to offer the support that their partners needed. Over and over again women's accounts of their birth experiences made it evident that a man's fears were quickly communicated to the woman, and that as well as having to cope with the challenges of her labour she had to worry about what he was going through.

In many cultures, however, his physical labour is needed to prepare the birth room and for the lying-in afterwards. In south-east Asia he may build a birth hut, or prepare bark cloth and make a bed for the woman's fire-rest afterwards, as on the island of Sarawak. He constructs a hedged birth sanctuary, or chops down a tree and saws and carves stakes, then sets them in the ground to support the woman as she pushes the baby out, as in indigenous cultures on the Great Plains of North America. If the labour is difficult he may be called in to confess adultery during the pregnancy, as in peasant Greece, because only such confession can remove the blockage to birth. He may be asked to give physical support, holding his wife in his arms and leaning her against his body. Or his presence may even be required so that a string can be tied round his testicles on which the woman can pull as each contraction mounts to a peak of pain, as in the Huichol tribe of Mexico.

'I will lift up mine eyes unto the hills, From whence cometh my help. My help cometh from the Lord, Which made heaven and earth . . .'

The father often has an important spiritual function. He speaks directly to God and prays for the birth to go well and the baby to be safe and healthy. He draws on the words of the patriarchs and the poetry of his ancestors. Both Moslem and Jewish faiths assign the father a strong spiritual role during childbirth. A Moslem father can help the birth through prayer. And all the men in a Sephardic Jewish household gather to pray when a woman is in labour, reciting Psalm 121: 'I will lift up mine eyes unto the hills, From whence cometh my help. My help cometh from the Lord, Which made heaven and earth . . .'; and Samuel 1 or Genesis 21, verses 1 to 8. In Germany in the 18th century the husband walked up and down in front of the door of the birth room reading Isaiah 54 aloud three times. If the birth was long and difficult he told the rabbi so that the Torah scroll might be brought from the synagogue and placed in the birth room. Still today the Orthodox Jewish father has the responsibility of sitting in a nearby room and reading the psalms aloud.

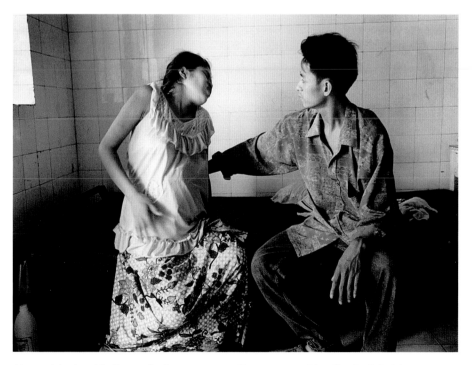

Above: A husband in Phnom Penh attempts to offer support to his wife who is in labour.

Doulas

Penny Simkin began to train doulas – women who give time to support other women in childbirth, not as midwives but as sisters sharing the experience – at the Seattle Midwifery School in 1988, because her research on the long-term impact of women's first birth experiences revealed that women remember their births vividly, and often poignantly, even twenty years later. Their level of satisfaction is strongly associated, not with length of labour, with complications, or whether they had drugs for pain relief, but with the way they were treated by those caring for them. In 1992 she started Doulas of North America, and now over 3,000 doulas are being trained every year.

The doula movement was slow to start in Britain. There are huge cultural differences in maternity care between Britain and the USA. Midwifery was virtually destroyed in America and obstetric nurses took the place of midwives, though midwifery is now being rediscovered. In Britain there is a tradition of personal attention and emotional support from midwives. In practice, however, when hospitals are understaffed and midwives are overworked and come and go on a shift system, women cannot get to know their midwives and care is fragmented.

In Britain, the first doulas were antenatal teachers who were invited by mothers they had taught to attend their births. From the 1970s on, many teachers and student teachers did this if a woman was without a partner, if a partner was anxious, or if past experience – the death of a baby or a dramatic birth for example – or emotional distress at the time indicated that they had special needs. This was discouraged by the National Childbirth Trust (NCT) because there was no insurance cover for the teachers who took on this role. Yet tutors considered it an important element in teacher training and valued the practical experience it offered. Many midwives welcomed these NCT students and teachers, but others were anxious that they were invading their territory and usurping their own role, that they might interfere in the birth, even that they could be spies lying in wait to report on malpractice and negligence. The trust and spontaneous ease that existed between midwives and home care assistants in the Netherlands was missing. A doula had to forge a relationship with each midwife, and when a midwife was concerned to stay in control and assert her authority, this was sometimes hard to do.

In contrast, occasionally the opposite occurred and a midwife entered the partnership gladly, but expected the woman companion to take on tasks for which she was not trained and could not accept responsibility, such as checking the fetal heart. The role of a birth companion needed clearly defining.

Doulas today focus on two phases of birth: labour and delivery, and the postpartum period. Some give care throughout this time, others only during birth or only postpartum. While the first training courses were set up in the mid-1990s, they did not get any publicity until 1998, when the media seized on the subject as highly relevant to the needs of women who did not have friends and family available during childbirth or to help afterwards.

Women most in need of birth companionship are those least likely to get it: teenage single mothers, the very poor and socially isolated, those who speak no English, and women in prisons. Probably the most vulnerable of all are women prisoners, who fall into all these categories and are also likely to be black. In 1996, a doula group was started for prisoners in Holloway Prison, London, the largest women's prison in Europe. These doulas, or 'birth sisters' as the prisoners call them, offer their services voluntarily for any woman who wants them, and have developed a special training scheme. A doula visits the woman in prison during pregnancy to discuss what she wants, meets her in hospital to support her during antenatal care if she wishes, goes to the hospital as soon as it is known that she is in labour, stays with her throughout labour and birth, and gives her support after the birth, including help with breastfeeding if this is her choice. One member of the group teaches the antenatal classes in the prison and has continuing contact with pregnant prisoners and new mothers. Another member of the group is a trained breastfeeding counsellor.

The mother of a prisoner told me afterwards, 'The birth sister was very good. I had forgotten what to do, it was so long ago I had my children. She walked around with her, rubbed her back, touched her, gave her water, breathed with her and encouraged her all the time. She was amazing! It was just like what the women do at birth back home in Nigeria.'

These women are a modern version of the god-sibs whom women in the past could rely on to help them. They do not take the place of a midwife. They provide loving emotional support and comfort, and in doing so increase a woman's self-confidence and free her so that she can let her body give birth.

Chapter 5

Midwives

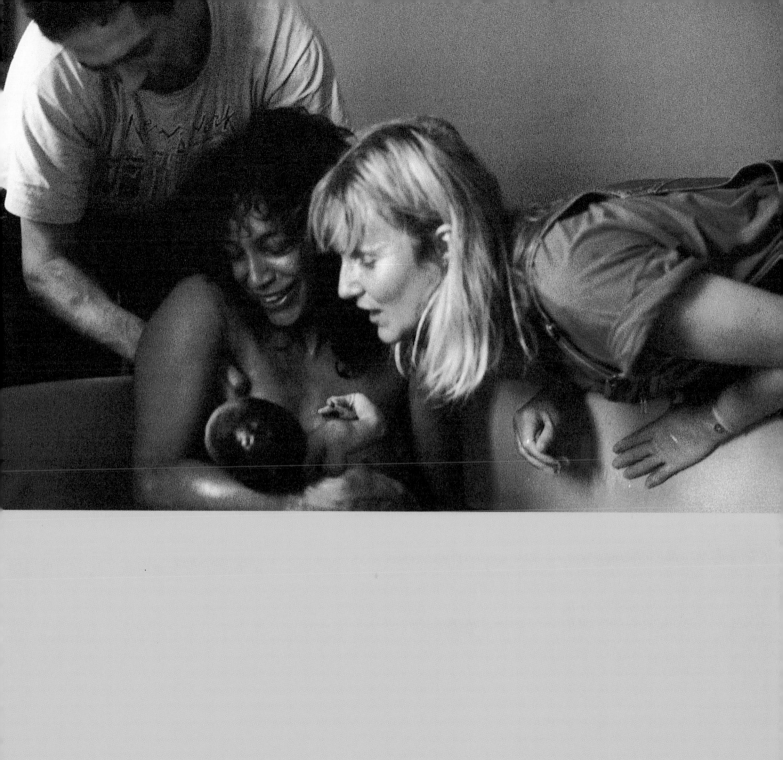

Midwife: a word that can mean many different things. She may be a trained nurse; a direct entry midwife with both academic learning and empirical skills derived from apprenticeship and personal experience; a 'lay' midwife, all of whose skills come from apprenticeship and direct experience, as are many American midwives today; a healer who also delivers babies; a young woman barely out of college who has never given birth herself; a grandmother or mother who has borne many children and helps women in her community give birth; or perhaps a woman with the knowledge to procure abortion and bring down women's 'courses' with ergot, pennyroyal, savin or other herbs, and who knows how to mix love potions.

She may be a highly respected authority figure, like a *nana*, the traditional midwife in rural Jamaica, who is one of a female triad – midwife, school teacher and postmistress – through whom all the politics of the local community are conducted, or a woman who is of low caste because she deals with the 'dirt' and pollution surrounding childbirth, as is the *dai* in rural India. She may have understanding of women's mysteries and the holiness of birth, or may simply be concerned to process parturient women through the hospital system. She may work alone, in a partnership, or as one of a team. She may be a friend or a complete stranger. She may even be a man.

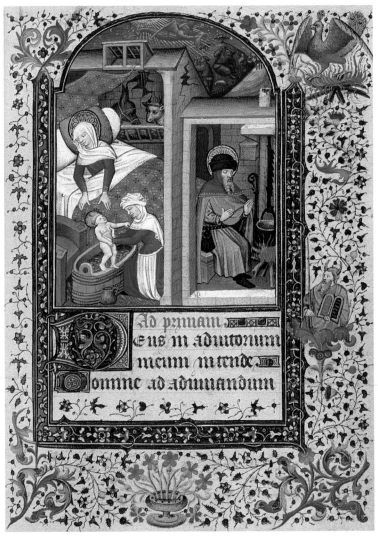

Right: A manuscript showing a midwife bathing the infant Jesus.

To be a 'midwife' means literally to be 'with woman'. The word comes from the old English. In other languages the midwife is the woman who places herself in front of the mother (Italy), the one who holds (Navajo), the earth-mother (Denmark and India), the woman who massages, the woman who picks up the baby, the woman who leads the child by the hand to be with us, the bathing woman, the woman who holds the pelvis and the woman who supports the mother from behind (all terms used in Japan), the wise woman (France), medicine woman (many Native American tribes), the cord mother (Inuit), and the grandmother of the umbilical cord (Nicaragua). In these two cultures the midwife has a life-long relationship with the child. She becomes family.

As we have seen already in exploring concepts of birth and the spirit, a midwife often enables a woman to draw on spiritual forces to give birth, rather than merely supervising or directing a bio-mechanical process.

In traditional societies birth is seen as an expression of health rather than sickness, and if anything goes wrong it is believed to result from disharmony. As we have seen, one important task of the midwife is to mediate so that there is social harmony. Anger or envy, unresolved conflicts, and infidelity by either of the parents can delay dilatation. The midwife diagnoses what is blocking the progress of birth, may guide confession, offer a prayer for forgiveness and suggest reconciliation. She may advise that a gift be given to someone who has been wronged, or, as in rural Greece, that someone who is angry with the woman who is in labour comes to her, bearing in their cupped hands water for her to drink. She has a spiritual function and also mediates between the physical body and divine powers. She may offer sacrifices to the gods, or call on a shaman to enact a psycho-drama that will dissolve the negative forces which are delaying the birth.

Traditionally, the midwife is a specialist in using symbols that have a psychosomatic effect, and is an expert in symbolic images of release that can open the way for birth. In ancient Greece, when a woman went into labour she untied the ritual knot of her girdle, dedicated to the goddess Artemis, so that her body might be similarly unloosed.[1] In peasant Greece today, doors and cupboards are unlocked to help the birth go well, and the husband undoes his tie and unbuttons his clothing. The midwife may suggest that water is poured through his shirt sleeves or down the chimney to symbolise the free-flow of life.[2]

In many other cultures, doors and windows are opened, corks and stoppers are taken out of bottles, and covers are lifted off containers in the kitchen while a woman labours. Grain is scattered and water flows.

In traditional Jewish communities, however, the emphasis is on security. All doors and windows are closed and locked against evil. In Eastern Europe, incantations to protect the woman against evil spirits, particularly Lilith, the winged female demon, were painted on the walls of the birth room and a circle chalked around the bed, while Psalm 121 was recited. Evil could not cross this line.[3]

A visual focus is often provided for the woman with an opening flower, which gradually spreads its petals in the heat of the room. This flower is called 'the hand of the Mother of God' in Greece. In peasant Italy it is the rose of Jericho. A similar practice is common in some areas of southern India. The unfurling petals symbolise dilatation of the cervix and the woman believes that as the flower unfurls so her body opens.

Spiritual power can be harnessed and concentrated in an object which represents creative energy. In Sri Lanka both Muslim and Hindu women wear an object made of iron during labour, for iron is powerful against demons.[4]

Among the Navajo a woman wears juniper seed birthing beads. Two straight bands of the seeds symbolise the rain, and a zigzag strand of bugle beads represents a journey on a road. A horizontal half-circle symbolises the rainbow spiritual path. It is this which links the child to creative forces.[5]

The Middle Ages

For hundreds of years in Europe the midwife choreographed the actions of the god-sibs. In this traditional role she did not exercise power as a member of an authoritative élite who possessed esoteric knowledge. Instead, she was one of a group of women who shared a common understanding of birth. She was acknowledged as having the most experience and understanding the prayers, charms and sacred acts that made birth easier – the massage and anointing, the movements and herbal infusions to deal with difficulties. She knew how to use the power of the word and the skill of her hands. Through words she produced images that overcame evil and gave women new strength. With her hands she could relieve pain, turn the baby into the right position for birth and coax the muscles of the birthway to soften and open. During my fieldwork in Jamaica in the 1960s, the *nanas*, the traditional midwives whose practices have their roots in both West African and European tradition, told me that their main work was to 'unstop' the woman's body and help it open freely. That, perhaps, is the essence of all midwifery.

An English midwifery manual of the 16th century, *The Birth of Mankind*, which went through eleven editions, describes the task of the midwife:

The midwife herself shall sit before the labouring woman, and shall diligently observe and wait, how much, and after what means, the child stirreth itself. Also shall with hands first anointed with the oil of Almonds, or the oil of White Lilies, rule and direct everything as she shall see best. Also the midwife must instruct and comfort the party, not only refreshing her with good meat and drink, but also with sweet words, giving her hope of a good speed in deliverance, encouraging and enstomaching her to patience and tolerance.[6]

Right: A manuscript showing witches worshipping the Devil in the form of a black goat.

This book was supposed to be written by a midwife called Trotula in Salerno, a famous centre of medical expertise, but was probably written by a man. There were few texts to consult, and many midwives could not read or write. A midwife learned, above all, from direct experience.

Through the 16th and 17th centuries in England, Germany, France and the Netherlands, local municipal authorities licensed midwives, but the proportion of unlicensed midwives was probably much higher. In England Quaker midwives were held in very high esteem. In Catholic countries midwives baptised any baby who looked as if it might not survive until the priest arrived, and had to work closely with the Church.

Members of the aristocracy often had their own celebrated midwives. As early as the 14th century, Asseline Alexandre travelled from Paris to attend three births of the Duchess of Burgundy. Jeanne La Goutiere was midwife to the Duchess of Orleans and is said to have gone as far as Bavaria to serve as midwife to Queen Isabeau. In England, Marjorie Cobbe was midwife to Edward IV's Queen.

Yet in the late Middle Ages midwives and the other women who helped at births were increasingly in danger of being denounced as witches. In the witch-hunts that occurred between 1560 and 1660 around 100,000 witches were condemned, 30,000 of them in Germany, and vast numbers, too, in Switzerland and France. Many, but by no means all, were midwives. Witches were usually elderly women who were disliked by their neighbours. They were often poor and were accused of being 'scolds'. A witch's curse could cause impotence, illness and the death of human beings and animals. In Britain it is estimated that two-thirds of accused witches were widows or spinsters. At the height of the witch-hunts the death of a baby or the birth of one with a disability might expose the midwife, especially one who was an elderly widow, to an accusation of witchcraft.

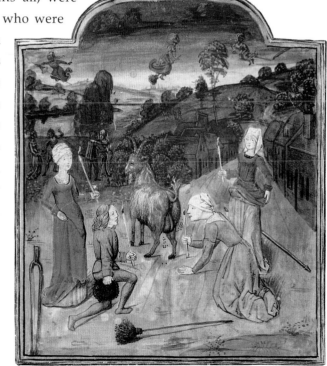

One characteristic of a witch was said to be a fingernail like a talon. Mediaeval midwives sometimes kept one fingernail long and sharply pointed in order to puncture the membranes, so it is not surprising that many midwives were tried and burned for witchcraft.

Early Modern Times

In many societies midwives have always been highly honoured. This was certainly the case with granny midwives who first arrived in America in cargoes of slaves from West Africa, and among those shipped to New South Wales in the 1780s and to Tasmania from 1820.

In Australia it was not only other female convicts who depended on their care, but all women. The discovery of gold in 1851 led to a tremendous increase in immigration to New South Wales, and the population had quadrupled by 1900. Yet in 1859 only nine women were officially registered as midwives.

Though in the early days women who were skilled at midwifery were allowed temporary release to attend women settlers in childbirth, in rural areas of Australia the granny midwife was an important institution. She not only delivered the baby, but cooked, cleaned and looked after the other children and the husband until the mother was fit enough to take on this work herself. She relied on her own mothering and management skills, and her midwifery techniques stemmed from empirical knowledge acquired from other midwives and vast practical experience in handling both straightforward and abnormal births.[7]

In North America, black midwives 'waited on' most births in the black community and, in rural areas, in the white community as well.

Margaret Charles Smith practised as a granny midwife in Alabama from 1949 to 1986, though a law making midwifery illegal was passed in 1976. She attended some 3,000 births and never lost a mother, and rarely a baby. Born in 1906, Margaret was raised by her grandmother, an ex-slave who had been transported to America from Africa when she was thirteen or fourteen years old and sold for $3.

When a midwife was working with a very poor mother she often had to help her in a shack with no running water. She made a palette out of torn quilts and rags on which she could kneel or squat. The County Health Department inspected the midwives' bags to make sure that they did not contain traditional herbs or any substance with which to

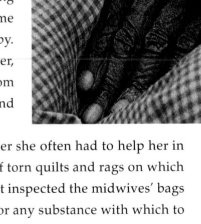

Above: The hands of an elderly granny midwife in Autauga County, USA.

massage the mother, because they believed it caused infections. So midwives kept two bags, one for use, with oils, herbs, roots and sugar and turpentine for healing tears, and another for inspections.[8]

In her final years of practice, Mrs Smith had to serve as an 'underground' midwife. After she retired she spoke out about hospital birth practices:

The nurse is the one who delivers the baby. They catch the baby. The doctors don't even be in there. Sometimes you have the baby by yourself. You holler and buck and rear until the baby comes. Some of the ladies, when they first started going to the hospital, they strapped you down and wouldn't allow you anything to eat. Right now, ladies going to the hospital say that often they look at you, feel your stomach then out the door he goes.

But these mothers, they still rather be in the hospital where they can whoop and holler thinking the doctor is going to give them something to ease them pains, but the doctors won't be here. The nurse be back there, and they come in there every occasions. You need somebody back there with you. Now a midwife, she has got to be right there, sitting right aside the bed or sitting over you, holding you, rocking you, loving you.[9]

Formal midwifery training did not start in North America until 1848. The Boston Female Medical College was opened because its founder was shocked that male doctors were seeing women's private parts and engaging in what he saw as indecency.

In Utah midwifery was strong because Mormon pioneers started midwifery schools around Salt Lake City in the mid-19th century. Brigham Young's wife was a midwife and delivered hundreds of babies, including more than fifty born to her husband's other wives. Some Mormon women studied at the Women's Medical College in Philadelphia and many went to work in other states, Arizona, Idaho, Nevada and New Mexico, where they were the only providers of health care.[10]

Male doctors objected to midwives because they believed no 'true' woman would want to do the kind of work that midwives had to do. Nor could women be trusted to think logically and make wise decisions because it was not in their nature to be calm, cool and reasonable:

They have not that power of action or that active power of mind, which is essential to the practice of a surgeon. They have less power of restraining and governing the natural tendencies to sympathy and are more exposed to yield to the expressions of acute sensibility . . . Where they become the principal agents, the feelings of sympathy are too powerful for the cool exercise of judgement.[11]

Not only were they likely to be overcome with emotion, but if it happened that they were menstruating at the time they might unwittingly kill their patients. Horatio Storer, a Boston doctor, wrote: 'Periodical infirmity of their sex . . . in every case . . . unfits them for any responsible effort of mind.' When women were menstruating 'neither life nor limb submitted to them would be as safe as at other times'. It was a state of 'temporary insanity'.[12]

Still in 1900, midwifery was unregulated in twenty states. While doctors attended more than 50 per cent of births, midwives cared for all the women who could not afford a doctor.[13] In 1912, the Federal Children's Bureau revealed that the death rate for American babies was higher than rates for most of Europe. In 1913, 15,000 or more American women died in or around childbirth and nearly half of the deaths were from 'childbed' or puerperal fever.[14] Women who gave birth in hospitals were especially likely to develop puerperal fever because doctors examined their patients without washing their hands. The cause of puerperal fever had already been discovered many years before, in the mid-1800s, by Dr Oliver Wendell Holmes in America, and also by Dr Agnaz Semmelweis in Austria, who found that the death rate of mothers from puerperal fever was three times higher in the part of the Vienna hospital run by doctors than in the part in which midwives worked.

A Professor of Obstetrics at Johns Hopkins University, Dr J. Whitridge Williams, sent out a questionnaire to all the medical schools in America which offered four year courses, and discovered that one third of the professors had no special obstetric training, one professor hadn't seen a single birth before he got his chair, and most medical students observed three labours or less throughout their studies.[15]

Williams could not accept the data. He wrote that the evidence 'seemed to indicate that women in labor are as safe in the hands of admittedly ignorant midwives as in those of poorly educated medical men'. But he decided that such a conclusion 'is contrary to reason'.

In the early years of the 20th century most midwives in the major cities of North America were recent immigrants. Many had excellent training diplomas from midwifery schools in Europe. In Sweden and Italy, for example, students had to conduct 100 deliveries under supervision before they could qualify. In New York City midwives assisted at 40 per cent of births, but only 22 per cent of births to women who died of puerperal sepsis had been attended by midwives. The vast majority of women who died of puerperal fever had been delivered by doctors. Yet in that study any death in which a midwife was present at any stage and at which a woman died was treated as a midwife birth.[16]

Midwives offered care after childbirth which was ' infinitely superior to the aftercare given by the average doctor for the same fee'. They visited the mother postpartum for up to ten days, cooked for her and performed 'little homely duties' as well as caring for the baby.

In the southern states and rural areas of the USA, women relied on help from 'granny midwives', now renamed 'grand midwives', many of whom were black. Until the 1970s, and sometimes beyond, these midwives served the poor white community as well as the black. Gladys Milton, a midwife in Florida, telling of her many years of experience said, 'In the space of a year, out of 140 deliveries, 98 of those were white . . . I believe I have about as much respect as anybody, black or white, in our area.' In 1985, she was one of the few grand midwives still licensed to work.

In spite of studies revealing the benefits of midwifery, midwives were forced out of practice and doctors took over. Wherever this happened more mothers and babies died. Midwifery became illegal in Massachusetts in 1907, when the maternal mortality rate was 4.7 per 1,000. By 1913 it had risen to 5.6 and by 1920 to 7.4 per 1,000. In the United States as a whole, as midwifery declined, deaths of babies from birth injuries rose by 44 per cent between 1918 and 1925.[17]

Meanwhile, Mary Breckinridge, an educated woman from a prominent southern family trained as a nurse, went to England to follow a midwifery programme. She worked as a midwife in the East End of London, and returned with some British midwives to set up the Frontier Nursing Service in Kentucky in 1925. In the first 1,000 deliveries not a single mother died. A report on the service revealed that if this kind of midwifery were available to American women generally, 'there would be a saving of 10,000 mothers' lives a year in the United States, there would be 30,000 less stillbirths and 30,000 more children alive at the end of the first month of life'.[18] Midwifery had been vindicated, but it was too late to prevent its erosion throughout the United States.

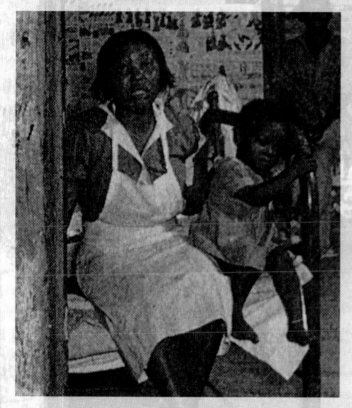

Above: A mother and child in their newspaper-walled shack in a southern state of the USA.

As obstetricians took over midwives were increasingly denigrated. A doctor writing in the 1935 issue of *The Alabama Medical Transactions* said, 'The midwife problem becomes more pernicious as the years roll by.'[19] In fact, in 1944 the *Alabama Medical Journal* recorded that neonatal mortality was 35 per cent higher for white babies, who were almost invariably delivered by doctors, than for black babies, who were delivered by granny midwives, and maternal mortality was 9 per cent higher for white women than for poor black women.[20]

In Britain and on the Continent most babies were still delivered by midwives. It was not until after the Second World War that they began to be displaced by obstetricians. Even so, in Britain today some 85 per cent of babies are still delivered by midwives. But midwifery in hospital is very different from the midwifery of the past, when women gave birth in their own homes and midwives were treated with great respect. A midwife historian describes what happened in Nottingham in the 1950s when the midwife was seen cycling along the terraced street towards a house where a baby was due:

As soon as the midwife's bike appeared, I sent the young one two doors up to fetch the . . . cup and saucers. She was the only woman on the road with a matching cup and saucer . . . We all borrowed it for visitors . . . I would run and wipe the 'lavvy' seat . . . I had four boys you see . . . The old man would push his paper down his waistcoat and slip over the back fence . . . to next door, he was really terrified of the midwife . . . I'd be left to face the music.[21]

Midwives who attended home births always needed to adapt to the domestic environment, which they entered as guests. Family life had to go on. It was rarely just a midwife and her patient. Other children, grannies, the husband, the neighbours – all took part in the unfolding script of childbirth, and the midwife worked surrounded by a bustle of people coming and going, and sometimes the baby's father snoring on the other side of the bed. One midwife recalls how she 'was called at 8 in the morning to a labour . . . She was getting on. . . She'd called the neighbour and got back in bed beside her husband . . . He'd only just got in bed after being on nights . . . a taxi driver. . . She didn't want to disturb his sleep before she had to. . . By the time I arrived she was pushing. . . I delivered the baby with her husband in bed. . . He'd woken up by then but felt too daft to get out in his pyjamas'.[22]

Practical experience and hands on knowledge remained the essence of a midwife's calling in European countries until the 1970s, when an influx of technology and the reorganisation of maternity services combined with the introduction of the American medical model of birth to switch the emphasis to management skills and the recording and storing of complex data. The system changed from one in which the midwife had personal responsibility to one in which she had little or no autonomy within a rigid medical and nursing hierarchy.

Meanwhile, in North America, where midwifery had been criminalised in many US states, or was outside the law, as in Canada until 1992, the poor in remote rural areas still relied on midwifery care, while those who were well off had private obstetricians. Today in North America midwives can work only if officially registered, and in many states of the USA no system of registration exists. A midwife can be sued for 'practising medicine without a licence'. It is as if parents were prosecuted for teaching their children to read and write because only qualified teachers are allowed to do that.

Doctors are unwilling to work in many rural areas of the United States and Canada and have always clustered in cities where lucrative employment can be found. In Alabama no licences have been issued to midwives since 1976, so outlawed midwives have attended births as friends of the family. Then a law was passed proclaiming that assistance at a birth by anybody without a doctor present was a criminal offence. If no doctor was available the woman was compelled to give birth by herself.

In South America and other Third World countries midwives still practise in inaccessible mountain terrain and in shack settlements on the outskirts of sprawling cities. Yet few midwives are completely insulated from the obstetric colonisation. When reproductive technology 'miracles' are extolled by the media, traditional midwives lose confidence in their abilities and borrow elements of practice from the medical model – frequent vaginal examination, injections, antibiotics, uterine stimulants, the supine or a modified lithotomy position for delivery and episiotomy – which introduce new risks into childbirth. In Mexican hospitals there is a high epidural rate, a Caesarean rate of up to 90 per cent, a 100 per cent episiotomy rate with vaginal births, and routine use of oxytocin. Many villages have a first aid post manned by nurses and house officers completing their internship, but women prefer the traditional midwife who knows about pregnancy massage and has practical skills and understanding of birth. Forty per cent of babies are still delivered by traditional midwives. Yet their existence is not officially acknowledged.

As midwifery was reborn in North America, midwives cared for teenagers, the poor, native Americans and black women and those who were often at high risk. Now they do this outreach work less than before because in many provinces and states in Canada and the United States these women are not covered by medical insurance, and it is relatively affluent women who have chosen 'alternative' care who seek out midwives. Midwifery is in danger of becoming a middle class luxury, while the disadvantaged are left attending huge over-crowded 'factory farm' clinics in inner city hospitals where they often feel they are treated like butchers' meat.[23]

A law was passed proclaiming that assistance at a birth by anybody without a doctor present was a criminal offence.

Birth Time

The medical model defines childbirth in terms of three stages: the first stage in which the cervix dilates to ten centimetres, the second stage in which the baby is expelled, and the third stage, in which the other products of conception, the placenta and membranes, are expelled. Sometimes a prelabour phase is acknowledged in which the cervix is ripening, and occasionally, in Sweden for example, an intermediate phase between the first and second stage is allowed for, during which the woman has as yet no spontaneous pushing urge, though she is fully dilated, and when the head descends further. Thus birth is segmented into specific periods of time and the time taken for each phase is noted on a record sheet.

The partogram is a graph on which the progress of dilatation and descent of the presenting part is recorded in relation to the clock. Friedman established a norm for this process – the 'Friedman curve' – and labours in hospitals across the globe are now mapped in this way. A labour that is considered too slow is speeded up. If descent of the presenting part fails to conform to the norm the obstetrician decides on instrumental delivery or Caesarean section. The partogram is the basis on which labour is 'actively managed'.

In traditional cultures, midwives still define birth in social terms rather than by medico-biological processes, and the times of these social events are only likely to be recorded if the midwife is literate and keeps a diary.

In the 18th century, the sensations experienced by the mother were often called the 'grinding' or 'preparing' pains of the first stage, 'forcing' pains of the second stage, and 'grumbling' pains of the third stage and postpartum. However, in America at this time, the most important way of describing the progress of any birth was in terms of the attendants to be summoned and their arrival or departure. The midwife might be called first. The next step, and a sign of progress, was when other women in the neighbourhood arrived. Following the birth the 'after nurse' came. Four days after the birth there would be an upsitting. Later the woman would be fit enough to make her bed – a definitive sign that she was just about back to normal. And finally, after about a week, she returned to her household work. In Laurel Thatcher Ulrich's book, *The Midwife's Tale: The Life of Martha Ballard*, based on a midwife's diaries written between 1785–1812, she writes: 'Parturition ended when the mother returned to her kitchen.'[24] Even the speediest labour was part of a long drawn out and gradual process.

Martha Ballard was the mother of nine children, learned her midwifery skills by attending births, and first served as a midwife in 1778. She describes what happened when she went to a woman because her patient felt that labour was about to start: 'I helpt Mrs Lithgow make Cake and Pies and knit on my Stockin.' The next day Mrs Lithgow was obviously in labour and Martha continued knitting her stocking. At ten o'clock that night Mrs Lithgow gave birth to a son.

Women kept active through the major part of the first stage of labour if they could: 'Mrs Walker was sprigh about house until 11' and gave birth at quarter past twelve. Another woman 'was able to work till near sunset'. The midwife helped with household chores and baking and worked alongside her patient. At night she might even share the mother's bed.

My mother, who was a midwife, described to me how, as late as the 1920s, the first thing to be done on attending a birth was to make sure that there was a good fire and then warm the baby clothes and cot bedding in front of it. She sat beside her patient doing needlework, chatting between contractions and rubbing her back and encouraging her as each contraction came. She prepared soup and milk pudding, and perhaps bread and butter and an egg to keep up her strength. When the woman felt she must push she would rig a towel round the woman's bedpost, the brass knob on a metal bed, or on to a door, so that she could stand and pull on it as she bore down. Once the baby was born and the midwife had checked its condition and wrapped it warmly, the father was invited in and the midwife made tea, though sometimes a woman chose to have her husband present to hold her as she gave birth. Later, the other members of the family came in, and finally visitors were welcomed. Birth was a social occasion.

This is still the situation in home births almost everywhere in the world. When a woman is in domestic space, the pattern of birth unfolds in a way that can never happen in a hospital setting, however 'homely' the environment or attractive the decor. Mealtimes, the time children get up and go to school, the rising and setting of the sun, changes in the weather, light streaming into the birth room, clouds gathering, frost and moonlight, the familiar sounds of neighbourly talk, children playing, and in the countryside of cows, sheep or goats, and birdsong – all of these have a profound effect on the parameters of birth time. They can make a painful labour less distressing and a long labour much more bearable.

This different perception of time affects what the midwife does. She knits another row or makes another pot of tea. She is under no pressure to intervene unnecessarily. Instead, she watches and waits.

In Malaysia, the midwife's first act on arrival is to make the woman herbal tea. She then massages her abdomen using the same herbal solution. She prepares the room and places metal by the mother to protect her and the baby against evil spirits. Then her main task is to sit, observe, wait and pray. She burns incense and makes invocations to the gods. The intervals between contractions are filled with soft chanting and muttered prayer. An English woman who gave birth in rural Malaysia said that she and the baby 'dictated the pace of proceedings' together. There is a kind of timelessness about birth under these conditions.

Once the baby is born, the midwife severs the umbilical cord with a slice of freshly cut bamboo. Then she massages and binds the mother. But birth is not completed until the placenta, the baby's 'little brother', has been buried near the house. Priya Vincent created the Birth Traditions Survival Bank at The University of Central Lancashire.[25] She has lived in Malaysia and India and told me that she was never close to the land or natural cycles until her years spent in these cultures. She talked about the different perception of time:

Now I live close to these natural cycles I can feel my body adjust to them – the monsoon followed by cool nights and hot days and then the heat of summer. In Ayurvedic and Chinese medicine the microcosm of the body is thought to mirror the macrocosm of the natural universe . . . I can feel rhythms both outside and inside my body which have a time of their own in that they take place at a pace almost of their own choosing and although each particular rhythm is similar it also varies from cycle to cycle. Seeing the process of labour and birth in these terms is to see it as another natural cycle with its own time which will be unique for each woman. I feel sure that this is how traditional midwives see labour and birth and how time is perceived. It may be why breastfeeding, which needs the harmonisation of the cycles of both mother and baby, is not perceived as an insuperable task but rather just another natural cycle that needs to be supported.

Birth is . . . a journey for which the specifics cannot be projected . . . The task of the traditional midwife is to support the mother in this process giving her whatever reassurance she needs (physical, verbal, ritual), to give birth successfully.

Accounts of birth in other cultures constructed by anthropologists tend to describe what midwives *do* to labouring women, and the rhythms of birth may be missed. Perhaps this is because we have not been trained to observe pauses, inaction and spaces, or to see waiting and what T. S. Eliot called 'a lucid stillness' as part of the pattern.

In the technocratic culture of birth, in contrast, time is measured. There are clear beginnings and clear endings which are recorded on a chart that frames the physiological processes being managed. As a result, another dimension of experience is omitted and a false impression given of the midwife's role. Midwifery is explained in terms of activity and intervention, rarely in terms of inaction or actions that may appear to an outsider to be irrelevant to the progress of the birth.

In traditional birth practices, on the other hand, where the counterpoint of uterine activity and relaxation is basic to the physiology of birth and the traditional midwife echoes this neuro-biological rhythm in her behaviour, the positive effect of her presence may be as much in stillness as in action.

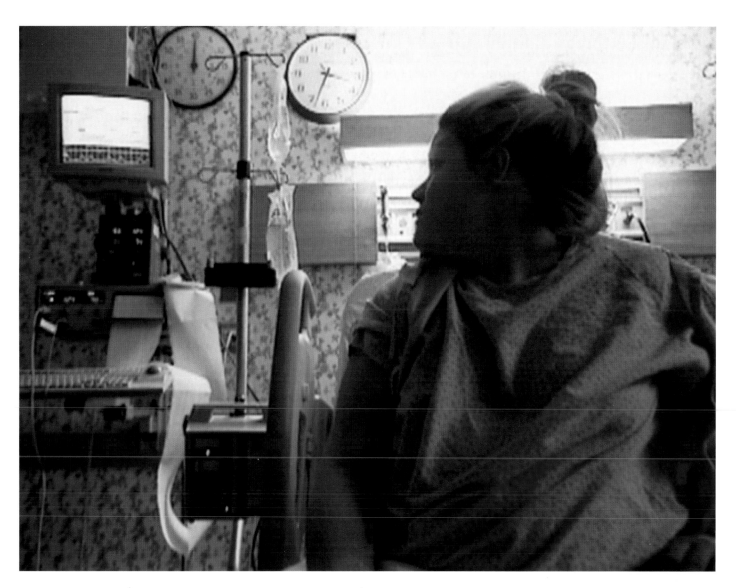

Above: The clock is the technology on which all the other technology used to manage birth is based.

The Placenta

If a placenta starts to separate from the endometrium (the lining of the uterine wall) but remains partially attached, the uterus is unable to contract evenly and squeeze on to the blood vessels so that they close. The result is that blood either leaks slowly and the mother becomes progressively weaker, or it pumps out in a massive haemorrhage and she dies within a short time.

When a placenta is partially retained in societies where manual removal or operative delivery and blood transfusion is impossible, the third stage of labour is recognised as hazardous unless the afterbirth arrives quickly. Though the baby is alive and vigorous, the mother's life may ebb away. Postpartum haemorrhage is the greatest single cause of death in childbirth worldwide, though reliable statistics on this are unobtainable.

When the baby is put to the breast immediately, nipple stimulation encourages the release of oxytocin in the mother's bloodstream; this makes the uterus contract so that the placenta separates and is expelled. But practice varies widely. In many traditional cultures the baby is put to another woman's breast or is given some other kind of fluid, because it is believed that colostrum is poisonous. So an important physiological protection against haemorrhage is ignored.

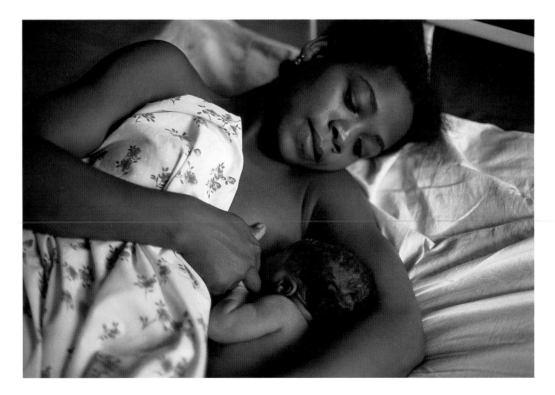

Left: When the baby is put to the breast immediately after birth, nipple stimulation encourages the release of oxytocin in the mother's bloodstream.

On the other hand, traditional midwives often delay cutting the cord until the placenta has been delivered. In South Africa a retained placenta was rare until birth attendants were taught to clamp and cut the cord immediately after the baby was born.[26] The advantage of delayed cord clamping and cutting is that blood flows from the placenta through the cord and thus reduces the volume of the placenta, so that it peels off the lining of the uterus easily. When a placenta is swollen with blood it is more likely to be adherent and the uterus has to work hard to expel it.

The World Health Organisation recommends active management of the third stage in countries where there are trained medical personnel. This entails the routine use of oxytocin. But it also recommends that where there are no trained birth attendants, and in countries where there is no safe transport and storage for oxytocic drugs, there should be research into the effects of nipple stimulation on oxytocin release and uterine contractility and on the timing of cord clamping on blood loss.[27]

Invariably in traditional cultures the placenta is treated with great respect. It is unusual for it to be casually discarded and it is often buried ritually with prayers and thanksgiving or, as with tribes of the Great American Plains, exposed in the branches of a tree until it is reduced to powder by the sun and wind. In the islands of Micronesia the umbilical cord is called 'the house of the soul' and is preserved in a small box or buried with the placenta – 'the friend of the baby' – near the homestead.[28] In America, the Cherokee father wrapped the placenta and walked with it over one, two or more mountain ridges, depending on whether the parents wanted the next birth to take place in one, two or more years, and then buried it secretly. If someone who wished the mother ill were able to obtain the placenta she could either be made infertile or could conceive again too soon.[29] In the Philippines, the placenta may be secreted in a bamboo tube and hung up in the house or on a tree beside it, where it will drive away evil, or in one tribal tradition it is placed in a jar and covered with bamboo leaves, since it has the power to keep the baby healthy.[30]

It is often believed that the placenta affects or foretells the baby's future. Because it is so powerful, a witch or a neighbour with evil intent who can seize it is able to harm the child at any point in its life. In some West African cultures a diviner may be called in to tell the child's future by studying the placenta.

Traditional midwives often have oxytocic substances ready to use in a third stage emergency. These include ergot, a fungus that grows on rye, which is the basis of the drug ergotamine, used to stimulate the uterus. Among the Zuni this is known as 'corn smut'. In the 1880s American doctors learned how to use ergot from midwives of the south-west tribes. Ergot was used by midwives in ancient Greece and Persia, too.

Midwives in other tribes used blue cuhosh, which they called 'squawroot' or 'papooseroot'. Mistletoe twigs, roasted over a fire, were also soaked in hot water to make a tea.[31] Mexican midwives may employ

Peruvian bark from the cinthona tree for its oxytocic qualities. Malaysian midwives give the mother a tea to drink in which is dissolved a powder from the dried placenta of a cat.

In many cultures the midwife tells the mother to blow into a bottle or hollow gourd. She takes a deep breath and continues to blow for as long as she can so that the muscles of her abdominal wall press in against the top of the uterus. It is undoubtedly a safer way of delivering the placenta than pulling on the cord. This practice is common throughout South America, in the Caribbean, among native Canadian tribes, in Sierra Leone and in the Philippines. Making the mother cough or sneeze may also help to deliver the placenta. Midwives in West and North African, Middle Eastern and Native American cultures use this method.[32] Or the midwife may make the mother vomit by putting the ends of her long hair in her throat or sticking a finger into it, a method practised among tribes of the American south-west and in Mexico.[33]

Heat is used widely. In Morocco, when there is delay in delivery of the placenta, the end of the cord may be placed in oil and heated over the embers. In some cultures the mother simply stands legs apart over a fire, a practice recorded in Malaysia and in native tribes of the western United States. George Engelmann remarked that sometimes Native American midwives made a steam bath. A hole was dug in the ground, filled with heated stones with fir tree leaves spread over them, and then water was poured over the top. The mother sat over the steam for a few minutes. He wrote, 'This simple means seldom fails.'[34]

The Midwife as Surgeon

In most cultures, midwives know how to keep birth normal. In traditional cultures when birth is highly abnormal they may be able to do little to help mother and baby and must rely on prayer and ritual acts. In high technology countries the skills of keeping birth normal are often neglected or trivialised.

Yet in some traditional cultures, too, midwifery entails interventions that damage the normal physiology of birth. Where female circumcision is practised it is usually midwives, and other elderly women, who perform the operation and it is the midwife who must open the woman's perineum with a razor blade before she can deliver, and who stitches her up again after. Midwives are so badly paid that they often depend on performing clitoridectomy (excising part or all of the clitoris) and infibulation (cutting the inner labia and part of the outer labia and stitching the sides together) for their livelihood. The practice is spreading in North Africa from Muslim to Christian communities. In spite of international concern it is considered necessary to ensure that a girl remains a virgin and is 'clean', 'pure' and genitally acceptable to a man. To be uncircumcised is to be dirty and polluted – *nigsa* in Arabic.

Pharaonic circumcision consists of removal of the clitoris and labia and sewing up the remaining tissues 'as tight as a drum', with only a minute hole left for passing urine and menstrual blood. A straw may be inserted to keep that hole open while the girl is healing. The Sunna version of the operation involves simply cutting the hood of the clitoris. Only a small proportion of girls receive this modified version of female circumcision. Most get the Pharaonic operation. It is practised in twenty African countries as well as in Oman, South Yemen, The United Arab Emirates and among Muslims in Indonesia and Polynesia. It is also performed on girls in Europe and America, and immigrants send their daughters back to Africa to be excised and infibulated.

The midwife in the role of surgeon, performing an unnecessary operation that leaves a girl genitally mutilated, is an anomaly in midwifery. Midwives may be under pressure to do this not only because they need the money, but because they are fearful that if they do not consent to it girls will have their genitals excised by others who do not use sterile equipment. This may result in chronic infections of the vagina and uterus. Sometimes the operation produces massive haemorrhage. Midwives know how to sterilise the razor blade, can suture with catgut instead of thorns to hold the flesh together, follow up their cases and treat infection with antibiotics.

Like Chinese foot-binding, European chastity belts and the Hindu practice of *suttee*, genital mutilation is an expression of women's low status in a society that is dominated by men. Midwives in such societies are often controlled by religious institutions which represent the dominant society, and though the midwife's territory is the domestic world of love and women, matters such as abortion and female circumcision are regulated by the dominant society.

Throughout large parts of Africa a bride who is discovered to be uncircumcised is likely to be rejected by the bridegroom, and the bride price or dowry must be returned. It might be thought that the practice would disappear as the standard of living went up. But this is not the case. When the economies of African countries improved, dowries escalated. In these societies women are the poorest and least educated and their status depends entirely upon making a good marriage. A woman proves her virginity through being circumcised, despite the fact that in the cities (where family members are unlikely to be watching over them as carefully as in the villages) women who have an affair before marriage can have anal intercourse without affecting the circumcision.

. . . the midwife's territory is the domestic world of love and women.

In the northern Sudan, 99 per cent of girls are circumcised.[35] The procedure is performed by women. 'It is precisely their dependence and material vulnerability that leads women to ignore the harm that attends female circumcision. Because childbearing in the context of marriage is the socially approved route to social and economic security, and infibulation renders women marriageable, most women . . . are still loath to risk their daughters' futures and continue to insist the procedure be done.'[36]

The anthropologist who makes this observation describes a birth in northern Sudan:

Sheffa tells Nemad to breathe; she wants her to cry out with the pain, rather than observe the custom of silence lest she hold her breath and deprive the baby of oxygen. A lamp is lit and passed to me through the window. I hold it high over Sheffa's shoulder. She inserts the syringe into the vaginal opening and makes several small injections around the area to be cut, much like a dentist freezing one's gums. Nemad is bearing down; Sheffa feels inside her and punctures the amniotic sac; fluid gushes onto the vinyl sheet and into a basin below. I fan away the flies. Soon the top of the baby's head shows through the opening. Sheffa pours water over the area to clean away some blood. She washes Nemad with carbolic soap then inserts two fingers between the head and the perineum. She waits until the head is crowning well, then quickly cuts through the muscle to the left and down. There is a spurt of blood . . . The flies are growing thick; hands rhythmically brush them away. After several more contractions the baby still cannot pass; Sheffa cuts a further inch or so. Next push, she eases back the muscle, gently grasps the baby's head and glides him into the world.[37]

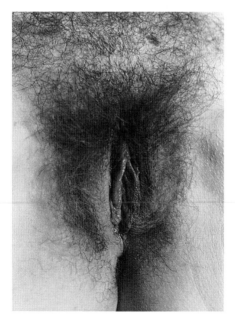

Within the medical model of birth that is now the norm in northern industrialised culture, and which is effectively colonising the rest of the world, a midwife becomes a surgeon every time she performs an episiotomy. This is an incision through the skin and muscle at the base of the vagina to enlarge the birth opening. It is either a cut straight down towards the anus (the usual practice in the United States) or a cut slanted outwards towards the buttock and then down in a hockey stick shaped curve (as in Britain).

Episiotomy is performed to hasten delivery when it is believed that the faster a baby can be got out from a woman's body, the better. So the midwife instructs a woman to bear down as hard and for as long as she can throughout each second stage contraction, and as soon as the head is on the perineum, or sometimes even before, performs an episiotomy.

Episiotomy was first written about by Sir Fielding Ould, Master of the Rotunda in Dublin, in 1742. He thought it was valuable when there was

Above: The perineum of a woman who has not had an episiotomy.

'delay in the birth of the head which, after it has past the Bones, thrusts the Flesh and Integuments before it, as if it were contained in a Purse'. He wrote that he would first try to open up the vagina with his fingers, but if that did not succeed he recommended making 'an Incision made toward the Anus with a Pair of crooked Probe Sizars'.[38] In those days it was an emergency operation which was rarely performed.

It remained so until the 20th century, when American obstetricians started performing episiotomies with enthusiasm. One asked, 'Why should we consider it other than reckless to allow the child's head to be used as a battering ram wherewith to shatter a resisting outlet? Why not open the gates and close them after the procession has passed?'[39] DeLee, who trained generations of medical students in Chicago, wrote in still more colourful, almost sadomasochistic language:

Labor has been called, and is believed by many to be, a normal function . . . and yet it is a decidedly pathologic process. If a woman falls on a pitchfork, and drives it through her perineum, we call that pathologic-abnormal, but if a large baby is driven through the pelvic floor, we say that it is natural, and therefore normal. If a baby were to have its head caught in a door very lightly, but enough to cause cerebral haemorrhage, we would say that it is decidedly pathologic, but when a baby's head is crushed against a tight pelvic floor, and the haemorrhage in the brain kills it, we call this normal . . . In both cases, the cause of the damage, the fall on the pitchfork and the crushing of the door, is pathogenic, that is disease-producing, and in the same sense labor is pathogenic, disease-producing, and anything pathogenic is pathologic or abnormal . . . So frequent are these bad effects, that I have often wondered whether Nature did not deliberately intend women should be used up in the process of reproduction, in a manner analogous to that of a salmon, which dies after spawning? Perhaps laceration, prolapse and all the evils soon to be mentioned are, in fact, natural to labor and therefore normal, in the same way as the death of the mother salmon and the death of the male bee in copulation, are natural and normal.[40]

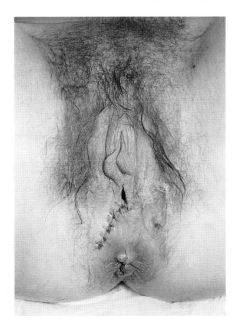

Above: After an episiotomy. She has had the British style cut. In the USA the scar would be mid-line to her anus.

This was not a new idea. Long before DeLee Luther believed that God made women disposable: 'If women get tired and die in childbearing there is no harm in that; let them die as long as they bear; they are made for that.'[41]

When a woman is commanded to push with all her strength and hold her breath for prolonged periods of time, and is not allowed to follow her instincts, her perineal tissues are likely to become thin and shiny. Episiotomy is then performed in the belief that it will avoid a tear. In fact, the most severe tears occur when an episiotomy has been done. They are extensions to the episiotomy. Just as any fabric can be ripped more easily once it has already been cut, perineal flesh and muscle is torn more easily following an episiotomy.

Episiotomy is the only surgical operation performed with scissors rather than a scalpel. If they are blunt, they crush tissues and nerve endings instead of slicing through them, with resulting bruising, granulation and nerve damage. Scissors are used to avoid nicking the baby's head. After the episiotomy the mother is stitched up. This may be done by the midwife, but in many countries midwives are not allowed to suture, or are discouraged from suturing because they are thought to be inadequately trained, and the process is carried out by a doctor. A junior doctor learns how to do this through practice. The first few times the only tissues a house officer has sutured may be those of a cut hand in casualty.

Obstetricians sometimes tell women that an episiotomy will avoid later prolapse. There is no evidence for this. Episiotomies may be performed because it is hospital policy to place a strict time limit on the second stage. The midwife does perform an episiotomy because she wants to help the woman avoid a forceps or ventouse delivery.

Like clitoridectomy and infibulation in Africa, episiotomy performed when it is unnecessary is ritual mutilation. It is the Western form of female genital mutilation.

The Midwife and Pollution

In many cultures a woman's body fluids hold danger for men. Male and female essences must be kept strictly apart. Menstrual blood, even the tiniest drop, threatens the male essence. If a man comes into contact with it he is made impotent or loses his strength so that he is easily vanquished in battle, killed by wild animals or drowned in the river. Even following the path on which a menstruating woman has just walked can weaken him. Childbirth is threatening to men because in giving birth the power of women's bodies is expressed in its most dramatic form.

Whilst this is likely to be distasteful or incomprehensible to many people in the West today, we may be able to understand it in terms of the way in which the Maori perceive women's bodies.

Among the Maori a woman's body is sacred, *tapu*, because it holds and gives life. In ideal terms, the female body imposes holy dread. The entrance to each *marae* is through the body of a woman and the carving above the entrance represents her genitals. Carved on the walls on a *marae* in Aotearoa, the spiritual centre of the Maori nation, are the words, '*He tapn te tinana O te wahine na te mea he whare tangata*': 'The body of woman is *tapu* because it is the house of humanity.'

In some cultures the work of the midwife is polluting. The *dai* in India has the same status as the female barber, *nain*, and the washer-woman, *dhaobin*, because they too handle the body and its products.

They used to be called 'out-castes'. Today, the politically correct term is 'the scheduled classes' and they are permitted to enter the temple.

Western thinking is dualistic. It is either/or. The opposite of 'pure' is 'polluted', the opposite of 'sacred', 'profane'. In Ayurvedic thinking categories are blurred, co-existing and merged.

Three worlds are involved in the process of birth: the 'nether' world which is contaminated, and the flow of substances from which defiles others, especially men; the 'middle' world that corresponds to the upper torso of the body; and the 'higher' spiritual world of the head and the brain. These three worlds are interdependent. The midwife understands and deals with the nether world and thus enables the whole organism to function effectively.

In a description of childbirth among Rajput women in Jaipur, Marcha Flint, a physical anthropologist, describes the role of Lockmi, a midwife who is a member of a caste stigmatised by ritual impurity.[42]

When Lockmi has been called to a woman in labour she washes her hands, removes her rings and bangles, and asks for help from the woman's female in-laws. They boil water for tea and heat up equal amounts of white glycerine and ghee (clarified butter made from water buffalo's milk) for her to use as lubrication when she examines her patient. With the mother lying on the swept bare floor, a pillow under her head, she dips her right index finger in the melted ghee and glycerine and does a vaginal examination. If labour is not far advanced she helps the mother walk round the room, leaning against the mud-plastered wall when she has a contraction, and massages her back using the ghee mixture. If labour is slow she offers her sips of tea laced with a herb which stimulates contractions, and may give an enema of soap and water. To further stimulate labour, the woman lies down and the midwife kneels over her, massaging over the sides of the abdomen with a kneading motion to the top of her thighs, her movements following the outline of the baby. Then the mother gets up and walks again, with the midwife always at her side, ready to massage her during contractions.

The author describes how the midwife straddles the mother and presses down on the top of the uterus to help her push the baby out. She goes on to say that in a very slow labour which had started at 3pm and continued until 11am the following day, with an interlude from midnight to 5am during which the mother rested, the woman suddenly motioned to her to help her get up and she delivered while the midwife was asleep. She wanted to be in an upright or semi-upright position.

Lockmi milked blood from the umbilical cord toward the baby, cut it and tied it with new string, gave the mother oral penicillin, and pressed on the woman's abdomen to deliver the placenta. This was then buried deep in the back yard under a mound of dirt so that animals could not root it up.

Lockmi inserted a little finger in the ghee mixture and stimulated the baby's anus so that it passed a motion. Then she took a clean rag and washed the baby with soap and warm water, lightly massaged it with the melted ghee, bound the abdomen with a rag and loosely swaddled the baby. If the baby was a boy the woman's mother-in-law beat a gong to announce his birth to the community. If it was a girl there was no ceremony.

She did not bathe the mother fully until the day after the birth, but washed her face, hands and perineum and changed her clothing. If there was excessive bleeding the midwife used the bark of the cottonwood tree soaked in warm water to check haemorrhage.

This traditional midwife has clearly incorporated practices from the medical model of birth and, as a result, care during childbirth is an expression of two conflicting cultural perceptions of birth.

Midwives and Taboo

Birth and death are situated at the perilous margins of life. Margins are places of fear and taboo. Anyone who lays out the dead, who embalms or prepares a corpse for burial, is working in that same place of dread. In many cultures midwives are called on to lay out the dead as well as to assist birth and abortion. They bind the corpse in a winding sheet just as they also swaddle the newborn. Dickens' Sairey Gamp attended deaths as well as births. She was a disreputable character who reeled between laying out the dead, placing pennies over their closed eyes, and catching babies. In his caricature of the midwife Dickens was expressing a popular stereotype – an old, raddled woman, very like a witch, who dabbled in blood, liquor, faeces and all the substances that cannot be contained as the body opens to give birth or to die. A nurse once told me that she had left midwifery because she found it distasteful: 'Bottoms, bowels and boobs.'

In gypsy culture childbirth is *mochadi* or ritually polluted. Menstruation, breastmilk, exposure of a woman's body, even the sight of her underwear; everything to do with birth is dangerous to men. In the past a woman laboured in a special tent and remained there for some time after birth. The tent, bedding and her eating utensils were then burned. This is why gypsies now choose hospital birth. Delivery in hospital prevents contamination of the caravan and the hospital midwife deals with a polluting act.[43]

Though there is joy in giving birth and welcoming a new life, women in cultures for whom the act of birth is pollution are socially contaminating, and the midwife who assists is soiled because she deals with the flow of fluids from the uterus and is in contact with the forbidden substances that come from a woman's body. So there is delight in birth, but at the same time dread of the female physiological processes that make birth possible. The spiritual categories of the holy and the dangerously polluting overlap each other.

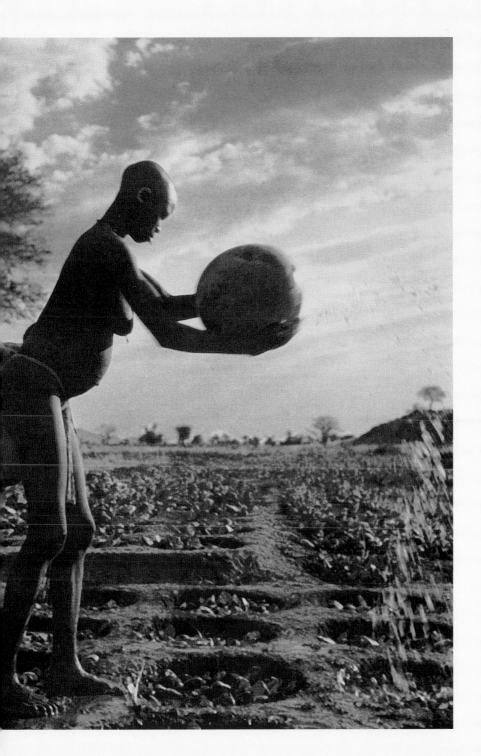

When Mothers and Babies Die

Women have been having babies since the human species evolved some 60,000 years ago. They have been amazingly successful at this. Yet birth is, and always has been, more dangerous where women live in poverty and are under-nourished, in countries where they bear heavy loads and have to walk vast distances to fetch fuel and water, and where the surgical skills and technology are not available to deal with obstructed labour. Whole families are shattered when a mother dies, for they depend on her labour in and often outside the home, as well as on the nurture she gives. Ninety-nine per cent of all maternal deaths are in the southern countries of the world.[44] Many are the result of botched abortion. In South America, for example, it has been estimated that up to half of maternal deaths are due to abortion.[45]

Left: Birth is more dangerous in countries where women bear heavy loads and have to walk vast distances to fetch fuel and water.

Discussion of maternal mortality purely in terms of medical management and research obscures wider social violence that makes mothers and children especially vulnerable. This includes lack of access to contraception, physical violence against women, sexual abuse, gender discrimination, malnutrition, the absence of roads, efficient transport and other means of communication – all these elements contribute to maternal deaths, even though they may seem to have little to do with childbirth. These deaths can be avoided only by social and political action and by raising the status of women.

Increasing medical resources will help up to a point, but does not offer a solution. Hi-tech hospitals eat up far too much of the health care budget. In some African countries hospitals absorb more than half the total health budget but only serve around 5 per cent of the population.

Introduction of the medical model of birth in Third World countries also results in the indigenous ways of conducting birth being downgraded and despised. Instead of a traditional midwife turning a baby from breech to a vertex position, a woman is transported to hospital for a Caesarean section. Rather than cutting the cord with a piece of sharp bamboo and then burning the umbilical cord stump with a candle flame, as traditional midwives in Yucatan used to do, they are taught to cut it with scissors. But there is a shortage of water, so the scissors do not get sterilised in boiling water and babies are exposed to the risk of tetanus. 'Low technology artefacts are simple, replaceable, interchangeable and easily procurable. Little prestige or commercial value attaches to them. Consequently there is no incentive for anyone to advocate their use'.[46]

The introduction of Western-style medical care in childbirth brings new risks. As the old knowledge is lost and drug, electronic firms and baby food manufacturers promote their products, these cultures are inundated with medical equipment, much of it outdated.

In Pakistan, obstetricians may be self-trained from text books written more than twenty years ago. Two English midwives who visited the Punjab to observe births in a maternity hospital in Sahiwal discovered that ultrasound was used freely and consulting rooms were 'all over the town'. All labouring women were given drugs to stimulate the uterus, without checking the baby's heart rate or calibrating the dose. As soon as a woman was admitted, one of her relatives had to go to the pharmacy to buy, at the family's own expense, antiseptic, a cord clamp, syringes, dextrose, an intravenous set, a cannula and three types of drugs.[47] Women had to labour flat on their backs on bare bed springs. Sheets were not changed between mothers and were only laundered once a week. Enemas were given routinely and frequent vaginal examinations with non-sterile gloves were performed, sometimes as many as three in half an hour. In the second stage of labour an attendant pushed on the top of the uterus with every contraction.

The former Director-General of the Indian Council of Medical Research states that:

It would be futile to erect a health care system based on the most recent and expensive technology without first applying proven ones such as those of immunisation, nutrition, sanitation and disease-free water. They were mainly responsible for the vast improvement in health that occurred in the 19th century and the early part of the 20th century in the industrialised countries.[48]

Maternal deaths are rare in developed countries. They are usually the result of ectopic pregnancy (when the embryo develops in the fallopian tube – a consequence of pelvic inflammatory disease), hypertension, pulmonary or amniotic fluid embolism in a complicated birth, or medical error. Statistics are hard to come by. Britain is the only country in which there is a regular 'Confidential Enquiry' into every death in pregnancy and childbirth. No such enquiry exists in the USA. But we do know that there, four times more black women die than white women, and black babies are twice as likely to die in the first year of life.[49]

In the richest countries of the world every baby is expected to live, and it is not only a personal tragedy but a terrible shock when a baby does not survive birth. One hundred years ago friends and family would say, 'The Lord giveth, the Lord taketh away.' Nowadays women ask, 'What did I do wrong?', 'What did the doctors do wrong?' There usually has to be someone to blame. At the same time researchers and clinicians ask, 'How can deaths like this be avoided?' A tremendous effort is put into discovering more about fetal development, the uterine environment, and ways of making pregnancy and birth safer.

Yet safe childbirth is not just a matter of medical care. The main reason for babies being born preterm or born at term but of low birthweight is poverty. Their mothers are the least likely to be healthy and the most likely to be badly nourished. Similarly, a baby whose father is an unskilled manual worker is nearly twice as likely to be stillborn or to die in the first year of life as a baby from a professional family. In any society where there is a gulf between rich and poor these are the babies who are most at risk.

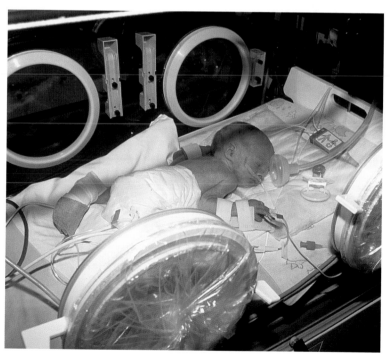

Above: A newborn baby in an incubator.

A Traditional Midwife in Jamaica

Though illegal in modern Jamaica, *nanas* are women of high standing and great authority in their local communities. The triad of the postmistress, the school teacher and the *nana* forms the political centre of each community, controls channels of communication within it and presides over the transitional rites in each woman's life cycle.

Channels for social mobility are very restricted in peasant communities and the two other positions of high status, the postmistress and the teacher, both entail educational qualifications. The *nana* role is the only one which bypasses formal learning. It overlaps with the ritual role of women in cult groups. *Nanas* are active members of churches and charismatic leaders in spirit possession. Most of the *nanas* I interviewed in the 1960s were central figures in their church and this gave an extra dimension of authority to their midwifery role.

The word *nana* is the same as that used for the 'grandmothers' who cared for the children of slaves while their mothers worked in the plantation. *Nanas* are grandmother figures. They are a link with the ancestors, shepherding between spirit and human worlds, and guarding the threshold of life and death.

The skills of the *nana* are handed down from mother to daughter. Nowadays this may mean that a daughter goes off to train as a nurse and midwife; nine of the eleven *nanas* I met during my fieldwork had daughters who were training in British or other hospitals overseas. Within rural communities, skills are assessed entirely by results and it is only possible for a woman to be accepted as a *nana* if the outcome for those in her care is good.

No-one can become a *nana* until she has had children herself. To be a *nana* is an extension of the mothering role, so all are mothers who are seen to be coping and successful in their role. Their social esteem is expressed by the term 'mistress', a title otherwise restricted to married women. They are also neighbourly women, willing to lend a hand, help out in times of family crisis, and, above all, are social facilitators. The first request to help at a birth is in the nature of a trial and if all goes well and her client likes her others will also engage her services.

There is conflict between the medical and nursing professions – pioneers of asepsis and order on the one hand, and folk midwives who do things 'the old way' on the other. If a woman haemorrhages the *nana* calls in the trained midwife and then poses as a relative, or sends the woman to hospital. Professionals believe that nanas produce haemorrhage, though since they only see cases in which there is haemorrhage this inference is probably false.

Attempts to incorporate *nanas* into organised health care have been met with suspicion by professionals. An epidemiologist taught traditional nanas how to weigh and measure babies for his study and at the same time showed them how to sterilise scissors with which they cut the cord. The *nanas* co-operated gladly, but he was accused by colleagues of trying to train an inferior category of health worker and the project was dropped. In the 1960s, around 50 per cent of Jamaican babies were delivered by *nanas*, though such births were registered as 'born unattended' or 'delivered by mother' (or by a friend or relative).

For a small payment in cash or kind the *nana* visits the expectant mother at intervals through pregnancy to counsel her and, using oil from the wild castor plant or olive oil, massages her abdomen and 'shapes the baby'. She usually knows her and her family before the pregnancy starts, but frequent visits mean that the two get to know each other very well. Most *nanas* do not charge the very poor. After the birth they care for mother and baby and for any other children of the family, and do the housekeeping, washing and shopping until the mother is ready to take over. In this they are assisted by the mother's female kin and the women work together in a shared enterprise in much the same way as did the god-sibs of mediaeval England.

The *nana* is the wise older friend who shepherds the woman and her baby safely through pregnancy, birth and the postpartum period. The bringing to life of the baby is seen as a process through which a woman needs to be accompanied, and though the birth is a dramatic event it is not usually perceived as a medical crisis. Women often complain to me far more about the discomforts and trials of pregnancy than any pain and distress in labour. The *nana* guards this passage.

Because the mother is in a state of transitional being and the baby is undergoing the same transitional process, she is in ritual danger. She can only be safeguarded through the careful observance of taboos. The most important of these entails strict separation of the principles of life and death, a rule that is common for many different cultures. No pregnant woman must look at a dead body. Though she can be present when it is lying in the 'booth' at a 'set-up' for the dead she must on no account set eyes on it. The younger the mother the more vulnerable she is. Her blood will chill to the temperature of the corpse: 'Your body get cold. Energy leave you', and this results in the death of the baby and also sometimes of the mother, either immediately or when she is in labour. Nor must a pregnant woman hold another woman's baby under the age of three months or the child inside her will die. *Nanas* sometimes smile over these prohibitions and pride themselves on being up-to-date. Nevertheless, they give tacit support to them and explained to me that, for example, the prohibition on using a treadle sewing machine in advanced pregnancy is useful because many women sit long hours over their machines and get severe backache as a result.

Pregnant women and new mothers and babies are vulnerable to *duppies*. These are mischievous spirits of ancestors and they live in the cottonwood trees. They can lay hands on the baby and make it sicken and die. Eclampsia is interpreted as spirit possession, the *duppies* having taken over the soul of the sick woman. So many pre-eclamptic patients had seen *duppies* haunting the ward in the public maternity hospital in Kingston that it had to be moved to another floor of the building. The *nana* tells the woman to eat oranges, plenty of *callalu* (a vegetable-like spinach) to enrich the blood, okra to make the baby slide out, since its slippery inner surfaces are thought to grease the passages, and to drink bush teas. Those recommended are 'bitters', in particular *cerasee*, which cool the blood.

Sexual intercourse during pregnancy 'nourishes' the womb and keeps the birth canal open so that delivery is easy. I heard a *nana* explain to a woman whose partner had left her that labour was difficult because she had not had intercourse during pregnancy and so was 'closed'.

Right through pregnancy, birth and the days afterwards a woman must be careful, deliberate, free from anxiety and from emotional extremes, active but not overworked, eating moderately and behaving with circumspection. When the *nana* takes a woman under her care she accepts responsibility for guiding her in this way over the bridge into motherhood.

Many members of the Jamaican middle class think of *nanas* as evil old busy-bodies who kill almost as many as they help and who are opposed to every benefit of science and medicine. They are embarrassing symbols of customs associated with slavery. Yet I met many labouring women in a Kingston hospital who bemoaned the fact that they were not in the country under a *nana's* care because they believed she knew how to make a woman comfortable, had better means of pain relief, encouraged her in a kinder way, and was able to make birth easier. Women often compared a birth in hospital with an earlier birth with a *nana* and felt neglected by professional midwives.

A basic Jamaican concept of ill health is that a passage or orifice is blocked. The cure consists of releasing the blockage. The *nana* sees her primary function as that of 'freeing' the mother's body for birth. Everything she does is designed to facilitate the natural process to 'bring on the pains in front', to let it 'open gradual', and to 'give them good words and cheer them up so that they will soon get deliverance'.

Nanas advise their clients to walk around during labour and the two women light the stove, fetch water and set it to boil, make the bed up with newspapers, tear up rags in which to wrap the baby and cook the cornmeal porridge which is the customary food for after the birth. During contractions in the late first stage, the *nana* massages the mother's lower abdomen, and in the second stage the perineum, with olive oil, castor oil or the oil from 'toona' leaves. Hot compresses are also used. She gives herbal teas, especially thyme, and spice teas for uterine inertia and prolonged labour. If the birth is delayed and a sweat-soaked shirt of the baby's father can be obtained, the mother is urged to take deep breaths of this to accelerate labour.

Nanas perform external inversion of breech babies and when there is a posterior presentation they use massage to rotate the head to the anterior. Some send the mother to hospital if they are unable to turn a breech; others deliver a breech, allowing the baby's body to hang by its own weight and raising the legs up over the mother's pubis to deliver the after-coming head.

To treat backache the *nana* uses a band of cotton cloth of approximately a fore-arm's width, which she extends round the mother's sacro-lumbar region and, facing her patient, pulls this cloth alternately from side to side during contractions to produce strong friction. If labour is hard she may wrap the mother in hot, wet towels, and when the skin is warm, remove them and massage her entire body with olive oil.

Nanas tell women to breathe lightly in the late first stage. It is believed that the baby can ascend into the mother's chest and 'by inhaling more the baby come up'. The *nanas* say this does not really happen but it encourages a woman to breathe shallowly and quickly: 'Too much heavy breathing gives bad sensations' (a reference to hyper-ventilation).

In the second stage of labour a helper or the woman's consort is often called in to support the mother's back so that she sits up for delivery, legs apart and feet on the bed. If other children are in the bed a washing line may be suspended down the length of the bed and a cloth thrown over it, separating them from the labouring woman; the nana delivers the baby up over the screen to show the children immediately.

Prolonged breath-holding and straining is discouraged, as Mistress Wilhel, an experienced *nana* who kept an 'accounter book' with details of more than 2,000 labours she had attended since 1927, explained: 'You push gentle and you give a little rest and you push again. Pushing hard brings on weakness.'

At delivery, the *nana* lies the baby on its front on the mother's abdomen and does not cut the cord until it stops pulsating, and often, in fact, leaves it until after the placenta is delivered. If the baby is not breathing well she holds the head down, 'milks' mucus from the nose by pinching the nostrils, and then blows cigarette smoke on to its anterior fontanelle (*mole*). If there is bleeding in the third stage the *nana* instructs the mother to take a deep breath and then blow into a bottle, which causes pressure on the fundus and tends to produce strong uterine contractions. The mother's vulva is cleaned by having her stand over a bucket of steaming water. The baby is washed in cold water tinted with washing blue to keep away the *duppies*, though modern midwifery practice has introduced antiseptic solution, which used liberally tends to produce skin rashes. The cord stump is treated with grated nutmeg (which has antiseptic qualities and is a mild irritant, so causing the cord to slough off early) mixed with powder, and a binder is put on. The *nana* massages the baby with coconut or olive oil and often gives a prelacteal feed of Jack-in-the-Bush or mint tea, puts three drops of castor oil on the tongue to make the baby cough up any further mucus, and then puts the child to the breast. She binds the mother's head in a turban to protect her against *baby chill* and puts the baby into bed beside her.

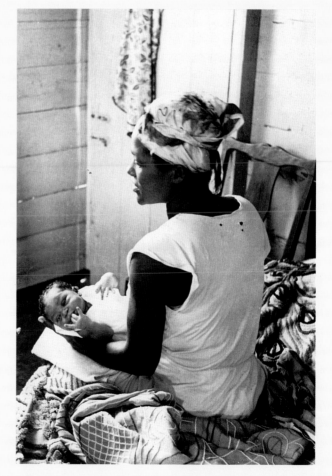

Right: A new mother in Jamaica wears a turban to protect her from *baby chill*.

The Death of Midwifery Traditions

The Inuit in the north-west territories of Canada are dispersed over 1.3 million square miles. Their land covers one third of the total area of the country. They live in scattered, often remote, settlements.

Until thirty or forty years ago every woman, and most men, learned midwifery skills, and knew what to do to help at a birth if they were needed. A woman might go into labour in a temporary shack constructed of sods or logs, in an igloo, while travelling by sledge, in a boat, or even in the open on a barren, icy, wind-swept plain. Knowledge of how to support a woman in childbirth was shared by all those who happened to be present. They helped the woman kneel or squat on caribou skins, and tied the cord with caribou sinews.

All girls were educated about birth in preparation for womanhood, firstly through hearing birth stories and then through practical experience as they attended births and learned exactly what to do. As they grew up they were taught how to turn a baby from breech to vertex, for example, and how to deliver a retained placenta by getting the mother to put her long hair in her mouth until she vomited, or by manual extraction. While in nomad communities all members learned how to palpate the uterus and could massage and rotate the baby into the right position for birth. In permanent settlements, as in Labrador, women with this expertise were recognised as specialist midwives.

Each newborn child had a continuing relationship with the midwife and the midwife was presented with the first piece of sewing done by a girl and the first animal successfully hunted by a boy. The midwife and the child she delivered still had special names identifying their relationship. In one part of Nunavik a midwife who delivered a girl was called Sanaji or Sunnageeq and the girl was Analieq. If it was a boy, the midwife was Agnaqutiq and he was the midwife's Angusiaq.[50]

Today, indigenous midwifery has all but disappeared among the Inuit. This is partly because when people converted to Christianity they considered traditional practices heathen, and partly because of concern over high perinatal mortality rates among the Inuit.

Even though they had no midwifery training, nurses, together with a handful of nurse-midwives who had been trained in hospital birth practices, were introduced into Inuit communities and women were required to go to the nursing stations (now renamed 'community health' stations) to give birth.

Since the 1950s, as the medical system took control in the belief that hospital birth was safer, more and more pregnant women were evacuated by air to deliver in large hospitals in Winnipeg and other cities. Initially this was for 'high risk' cases only, though it included all those having first babies. It was later extended to all women. Around three weeks before her due date a woman is flown south to wait in bed and breakfast accommodation for labour to start, and to have it induced if the baby does not arrive when expected. Anxious about their children left at home, mothers become bored and depressed and many turn to alcohol and other drugs to find relief from stress.

Women also say that they do not like the way that they have to give birth in hospital. They are forced to deliver in a supine position instead of an upright one, which was part of their tradition, and also describe being tied up while giving birth. Many women say that children who have been born in hospital are different and no longer fit into the Inuit lifestyle.[51] There is a general feeling that babies born this way, outside their own communities, are not true Inuit. They have, in effect, been disinherited.

Several new birth centres have now been created and nurse-midwives are bringing in traditional midwives as assistants during childbirth, training some Inuit midwives to work alongside them, and at the same time learning some of the old Inuit ways themselves.

One pilot birthing project is in the Central Arctic Region of Keewatin at Rankin Inlet. It was opened in 1993 because it had an airstrip, an evacuation plane, a resident physician and the highest number of pregnant women in the region.[52] Here, traditional midwives are 'consultants' to the unit and some traditional practices, such as upright positions for birth, the use of herbs to stop haemorrhage, ways of caring for the newborn, and support for breastfeeding, have been reintroduced. This is taking place alongside a control group of women in another Keewatin community who receive antenatal care from nurses, rather than midwives, and who continue to be evacuated to a hospital in the south to give birth.

The Best of the Old, The Best of the New: Bali

Bali is a crucible in which modern midwifery, Dutch style, has been combined smoothly and easily with traditional practices. Professional midwifery schools were set up by the Dutch in Indonesia in the 1920s. But after Indonesia's Declaration of Independence, the birth culture started to change to the American model, and the government stopped direct-entry midwifery training and made midwifery an extension of nurse training, with an extra year of study added. These nurse-midwives, the *bidans*, worked only in hospitals and did not want to practise in the countryside. As a result, traditional midwives, the *dukuns*, or 'medicine women', attended most births in rural areas, while in the towns nurse-midwives became assistants to male doctors. There was a sharp decline in the number of midwives in independent practice during the 1980s, and during this time the death rates for mothers and babies rose. However, good things were happening, too, because at the end of the 1970s a Balinese monk who was also an obstetrician, Dr Manuabe, set up a midwifery school which still flourishes.

Now the American medical model of birth has been rejected and the birth culture is similar to that of the Netherlands, but with traditional midwives working alongside professional midwives. In the northern province of Buleleng, for example, there are 20,000 births a year. Only 10 per cent of these women are delivered by an obstetrician. Sixty per cent are delivered by a *bidan*, 40 per cent of these in the *bidan's* home, 10 per cent in the mother's home, and 10 per cent at the local hospital. Thirty per cent of all women are still attended by a *dukun* at home.

The traditional midwife's work is holy and she is called to her vocation by the gods. Most *dukuns* register with the Midwives' Association, which organises twice yearly courses for them and sets up refresher workshops. Every month a professional midwife visits and supervises each *dukun*.

Dukuns and *bidans* work harmoniously together and relations with obstetricians are positive, too. If a *dukun* runs into difficulties she knows she can bring in the neighbourhood *bidan*. There are also small health centres where primary care for a number of villages is given, and midwives work a few days each month there, too, offering advice on health, family planning and nutrition and providing immunisation and antenatal care. In addition, there is a system of maternity assistants like that in the Netherlands.

Midwives are up-to-date with research and only introduce new practices when there is clear clinical evidence of their effectiveness. Antenatal care is meticulous. Beatrijs Smulders and Petra Blokker, both experienced Dutch midwives, make twice yearly visits to the northern province. They have done a great deal to help Balinese midwives. Beatrijs was present at a birth when a woman haemorrhaged and says:

Midwife Mila asked her maternity assistant to put two bricks under the legs of the woman's delivery bed so that Nyoman came to lie in the Trendelenburg position. She asked me to take her blood pressure. Before I had done so, I saw out of the corner of my eye how she had expelled the placenta as quick as a flash while her other hand supported the uterus. Her assistant stood ready with a syringe of syntometrine. The young mother suffered no ill effects. Myself – I had hardly noticed as she did it so quickly and routinely.

Most *dukuns* do not perform vaginal examinations. One says she gives only 'love and words' to help the baby come. Ketut Mastadi is a 65-year-old *dukun* who lives in a bamboo and straw cottage with very little furniture. Her delivery kit contains sterile scissors, a small bottle of alcohol to clean the cord stump, cotton wool and gauze, scales to weigh the baby, and because she is literate, unlike some other *dukuns*, a notebook in which she records the birth details. Ketut Mastadi visits a pregnant woman three or four times to give her strengthening herbs and massage. She prays for a good birth and the reincarnation of an ancestor in the baby and asks the gods to bless the baby. During labour she does not encourage any active pushing until she sees that the baby's head is pressing out the woman's anus, so that the second stage can be gentle and unforced.

The Midwives' Association borrows at low interest from the World Bank and can help midwives financially, enabling them to set up a practice, obtain equipment or buy a moped on which to get about. It also organises a ceremony every year, providing an opportunity for all the midwives to gather together. Each wears a beautiful, flowery sarong – the midwife's uniform.

The present-day birth culture in Bali is a success. The midwife has maintained her autonomy, traditional midwifery is respected, one-to-one care is the norm, women can still give birth in their own homes or their midwife's home, and hospital care and obstetric skills are available for any woman who needs them.

America and Britain

In the United States there are 34,000 obstetricians and only 9,000 midwives, 6,000 of them nurse-midwives and 3,000 direct-entry midwives. Obstetricians deliver 95 per cent of all babies. Many obstetricians fear competition from midwives, see them as a financial threat, and are determined to defend medical territory. Nurse-midwives train as nurses first and then go on to one or two years of hospital midwifery. Most of them work in hospitals under the direction of obstetricians.

In Britain, in contrast, there are 25,000 practising midwives and only 3,000 obstetricians. Through the National Health Service midwives provide the basis and substance of all maternity care; if they went on strike obstetricians would be unable to work after only an hour or so.

In North America there is ongoing debate between nurse-midwives and non-nurse-midwives about the necessary qualifications for midwifery, and how midwives work with the medical system. Those who are not nurses used to be called 'lay' or 'empirical' midwives, but are now usually called 'direct-entry' midwives. In the USA and Canada, the professionalisation of midwifery and its grudging acceptance by the medical system has led midwives whose skills derive from apprenticeship and practical experience to be marginalised unless they pass and work under the direction and according to the rules of big institutions. The American College of Nurse Midwives and the Midwifery Association of North America are struggling to work together, but there are many obstacles in the way.

In New York City, for example, nurse-midwives have at last gained the right to practise, but direct-entry midwives are required to take an academic course which is able to accommodate only very restricted numbers of new entrants. So they are effectively barred from practising legally. Nurse-midwives themselves are not happy about this. They want to move away from being defined as nurses towards greater autonomy. So in this respect at least nurse-midwives and direct-entry midwives have a common cause.

The conflict between nurse-midwives and direct-entry midwives does not exist in European countries. Midwives are midwives and they all work together, some in the community, some in hospitals, and many both in hospitals and communities. For European midwives the challenge comes in their relationship with obstetricians, junior medical staff and the medical system as a whole. In the

Netherlands, as in New Zealand, there is competition between midwives and general practitioners to care for women in childbirth. Family doctors often provide this service and many want to continue it. In Britain, however, general practitioners are rarely interested in attending birth, because it is inconvenient and badly paid. They prefer to offer antenatal and postpartum care only, and in effect much of this work is done by midwives attached to their practices, though it is still called 'general practitioner care'.

Many midwives want to offer continuity of care for all women and are highly critical of the segmented care provided at present. They gain job satisfaction from getting to know a woman during pregnancy, being with her in childbirth and caring for her afterwards. So there is a move towards midwifery group practices and one-to-one projects.[53]

In a meta-analysis of the organisation of midwifery care, Josephine Green and Mary Renfrew write that while some midwives find this the most satisfying way to work, others are concerned that their private lives will be destroyed by being 'on call'.[54] The debate among midwives continues.

In all cultures the midwife's place is on the threshold of life, where intense human emotions – fear, hope, longing, triumph and incredible physical power – enable a new human being to emerge. Her vocation is unique.

The art of the midwife is in understanding the relationship between psychological and physiological processes in childbirth. Rather than being the provider of a technical service to support a doctor, or someone who scuttles around getting ready for an obstetrician and clearing away after him, her skills lie at the point at which the emotional and biological touch and interact. She is not a manager of labour and delivery. Rather, she is the opener of doors, the one who releases, the nurturer. She is the strong anchor when there is fear and pain; the skilled friend who is in tune with the rhythms of birth, the mountain tops and chasms, the striving and the triumph.

Many midwives want to offer continuity of care for all women and are highly critical of the segmented care provided at present.

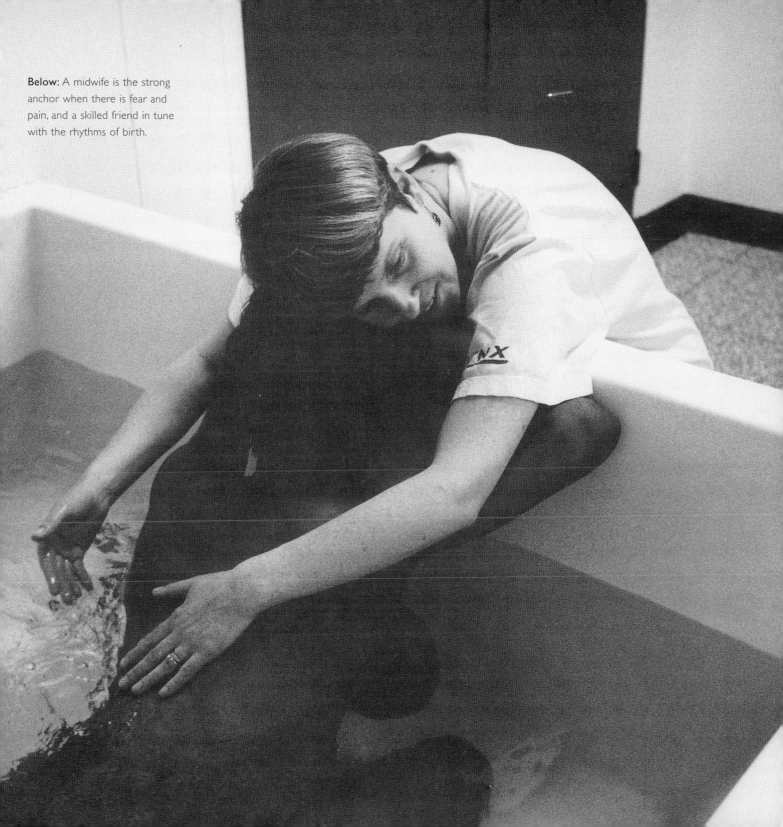

Below: A midwife is the strong anchor when there is fear and pain, and a skilled friend in tune with the rhythms of birth.

Chapter 6

The Birth Dance

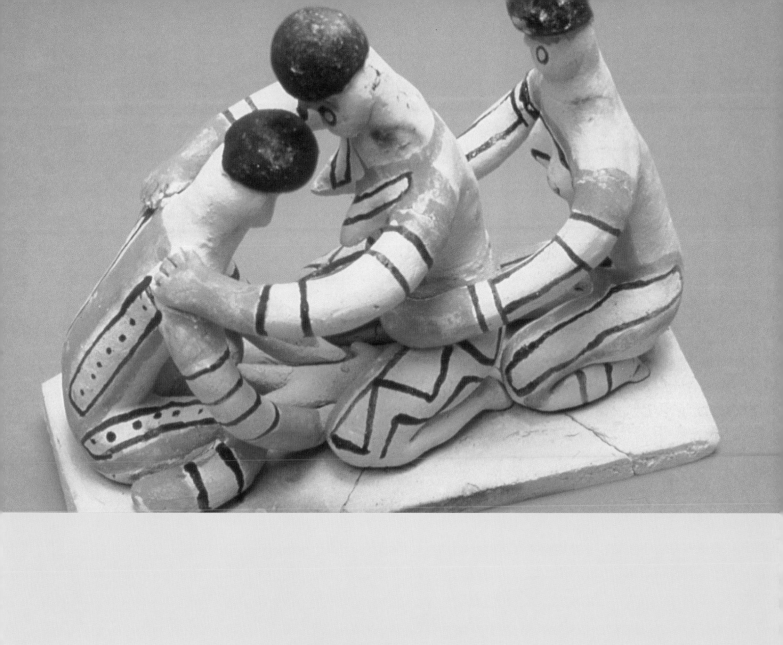

Everything women do in childbirth, and everything other people do to them, is profoundly affected by the setting in which birth takes place. Spontaneous behaviour and freedom to move depends on an environment in which a woman is not constrained or inhibited. She needs to be able to control the birth territory. In northern industrialised cultures today the majority of women are given little or no choice: it is hospital. Though they may have a choice of hospitals, home birth is out of the question. The only country in which hospital birth is not the norm is the Netherlands, where one-third of births still take place at home.

The Birth Place

Maternity hospitals were first established as charities for the indigent poor and unmarried women who were giving birth in sin. They were used as teaching institutions to train doctors. As early as the 17th century the Hotel Dieu in Paris was set up as a hospital where women could obtain free care. The medicalisation of birth entailed using destitute and working class women as demonstration material. In large cities across America and Western Europe, charity hospitals provided a rich supply of experimental subjects. In America many of them were black women.

The move from home to hospital took place first in the USA. By 1939 more than 75 per cent of births were in hospital and by 1960 close on 100 per cent. It did not make birth safer. The major cause of death was still sepsis.

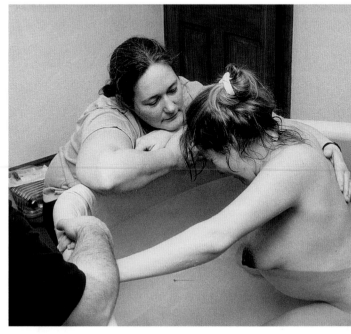

Even after the introduction of sterile procedures and the invention of antibiotics, cross-infection remains a problem in hospitals today, especially following instrumental delivery and other invasive procedures, though fortunately it is unlikely to cause death. Pelvic infection is one of the most common side-effects of Caesarean section. But all interventions, including simple vaginal examinations, increase the chance of infection. Women can usually withstand bacteria in their own homes. It is a different matter in hospital. Infection is a major concern in Eastern Europe and the Russian Federation, where a highly medicalised birth environment and rigid medical procedures are mandatory in the hope of avoiding it.

Deciding on a birth place is not only a matter of making decisions about *risk*. It has to do with *experience*, with how

Right: Being able to move freely and spontaneously depends on the birth environment.

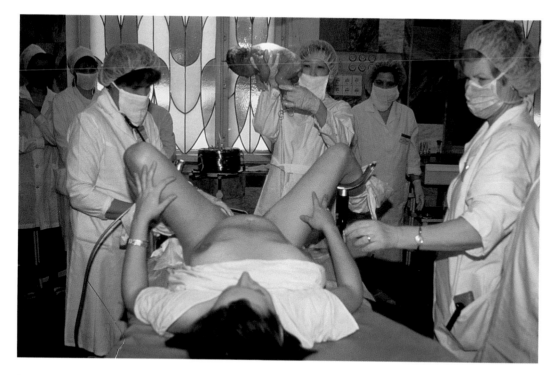

Right: Being able to move freely and spontaneously depends on the birth environment.

Below left: When a woman gives birth at home she is free to move, and has control over what is happening to her.

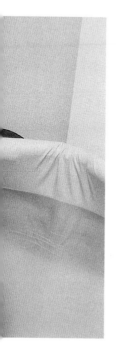

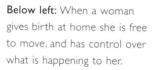

birth is lived and how it is remembered. One important aspect is a woman's sense of control, or her inability to control, what is happening to her, her sense of autonomy or constraint.[1] In the past, and still today in societies where a hospital system is not established or hospitals are inaccessible, birth has invariably taken place in domestic space that is under the control of women.

Native American women often laboured and delivered in the open air. Comanche women gave birth out of doors in a leafy shelter built by the woman's husband and well away from the camp. During labour the woman walked between vertical stakes he had set into the ground so that she could grasp them, bending her knees during contractions, and moving nearer and nearer to the secluded birth nest as her cervix dilated, in what was literally a journey to birth.

Plains Indian women often gave birth outside the *tepi* on a carpet of soft hay, leaning in front of a horizontal bar, with two heavy women or strong men sitting at either end to steady it so that the labouring women could grasp it without fear of it moving. The pushing bars sometimes fitted on to modern hospital beds are used in a similar way and enable women to bear down during childbirth.

Slave women in the Caribbean often gave birth in the open, too. Beside each sugar plantation was a tree known as the 'birth tree', and when at last a woman had to interrupt her work in order to give birth, she and two women helpers would leave the long line of slaves cutting sugar cane and go to the birth tree. There she would kneel or squat with her arms around the trunk, the women supporting her.

The Australian Aboriginal mother gave birth on a carpet of soft gum leaves, and women who were among the first colonists of Australia and lived in tents in isolated areas were often helped by an Aboriginal woman to give birth in the same way.

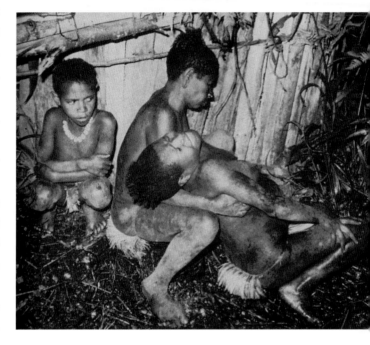

Maori women went into the bush with their helpers and made a nest called a *kourama*, lined with flax fibres to keep it warm. In one tribe it was the custom to give birth in the reeds by the river.

In New Guinea, the birth place is a small clearing in the forest, where the woman can crouch on a soft bed of creepers. A woman in central Africa might give birth out of doors sitting on a skin placed over a mound of sand. The sand slopes down to two stakes driven into the ground against which she can push with her feet, with other women supporting her back. The sand moulds itself to her body and supports her perineum. Sometimes, instead of a woman supporting her back, another firm mound of sand does so.

In all cultures in the past, a woman has either gone home to her mother and given birth there, as in Japan, or has given birth in the village where she lives with her husband, usually, though not always, in her home.

Even when hospitals were established they were often so far away that getting to one entailed a long and perilous journey. When Western Australia was colonised in the 19th century, for example, it was customary for the midwife to move into the mother's home and to live there with her until she no longer needed help after the baby's birth – often many weeks later. Sometimes it was more convenient for the mother to move into the midwife's house. For women in the Alice Springs area the alternative was horrendous: they would have to travel over 300 miles by buggy, horse or camel to Queensland, a journey which took six weeks, often encountering dust storms which were particularly dangerous on the return journey, because the baby might suffocate with the dust.[2]

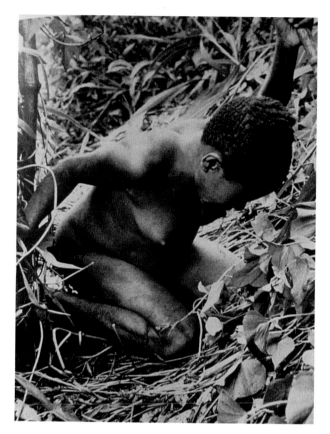

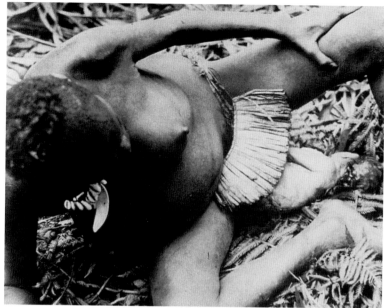

Above and left: In New Guinea the birth place is a small clearing in the forest, where the woman crouches on a soft bed of creepers.

In the Middle East a woman might give birth in the women's bath house; in parts of Africa in the menstrual hut, a familiar place where women rested when they had their periods, because there was a taboo against them cooking food for their men at that time; or, as in Sierra Leone, in the hut where a girl had been initiated in her mother's village.

In southern Africa birth takes place in the woman's grandmother's or her husband's grandmother's hut, because this is considered the safest place in the *kraal*. This is the abode of the ancestors and they will bless the birth. Moreover, if the grandmother is past the menopause her hut is uncontaminated by menstrual blood.[3] The Zulu woman also gives birth in a special hut, which has been prepared and decorated with beautiful objects and wood carvings, by girls who are virgins. It is believed that the first thing the baby sees must be beautiful. Every Zulu hut is constructed with a hole in the roof in order to maintain contact with the Great God who dwells in the heavens. As she labours the woman focuses on the little bit of sky that she can see through this hole, and it is said of one who gives birth at night that 'she counts the stars with pain'.

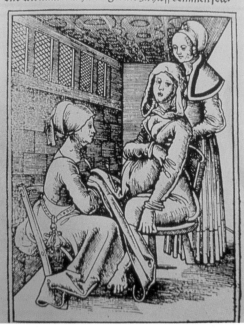

Right: The traditional birthing stool resembled the milking stool that the woman used in her cow shed.

A woman used to construct her own birth hut in rural areas of Japan, and birth took place in dim light, because the coming of the soul needed darkness and spiritual energy. A book that is half fable, half history, *The Kojiki*, written in 712, tells how the daughter of the Sea God, Her Augustness-Luxuriant-Jewel-Princess, built her birth hut where the waves met the sea-shore and used cormorant feathers for thatch.

The essence of a birth place is that a woman labours in territory which she, together with her women helpers, controls herself. She kneels or leans against ordinary household objects. She sits in a hammock, legs spread wide and hanging down at either side while she grasps another hammock that is suspended above her, as in Brazil. She crouches on a simple birth stool that has been brought by the midwife, which looks much like the milking stool the woman uses in her cow shed. She is supported in her bed by a bank of huge feather pillows; pulls on a rope hung from the rafters, as in Colonial America; or is propped against, or leans over, a bag of rice or a futon, as in Japan until American obstetrics were introduced after the Second World War. She kneels on two or three bricks, the traditional birth position in Egypt and some Middle Eastern countries. Or, as an elderly Chinese woman told me when describing the way she gave birth, she sits on a large wooden bowl with handles that she can grip when pushing. There is no specialised equipment, just comfortingly familiar objects which the woman uses every day.

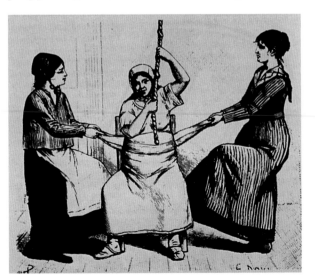

Left: A labouring woman in Colonial America pulls on a rope hanging from the rafters, with a woman on either side alternately pulling a strip of cloth above her fundus.

The choreography of birth in hospital presents a complete contrast to that typical of traditional patterns of care. The birth process is treated as a sequence of distinct phases, each conducted in a different room and managed by different professionals. This type of management was standard in the USA in the 1970s, and remains so in Eastern European countries. It is called 'three room' delivery.

The first stage of labour is conducted in a labour ward. Then the patient is moved to the delivery room where the baby is born, and from there to the recovery room. Transition from labour to delivery room takes place only after an obstetrician has performed a pelvic examination and declared that the cervix is fully dilated. Even when the woman cannot help pushing she must not be moved until official permission has been announced by the appropriate member of staff, and she is not considered to be in second stage until it is recorded on her chart. Until that ceremony is performed she is instructed not to push and a nurse may even grasp her knees forcibly together to prevent the baby's head emerging.

In modern hospitals these rooms are close to each other. In an old hospital, however, the woman might be wheeled the length of a corridor to get from one to the other. I have been in a hospital in northern Italy where patients had to be wheeled – often rushed – from the labour to the delivery room across a vast, echoing palatial hall to the other side of the building before they were allowed to give birth.

The birth process is treated as a sequence of distinct phases, each conducted in a different room and managed by different professionals.

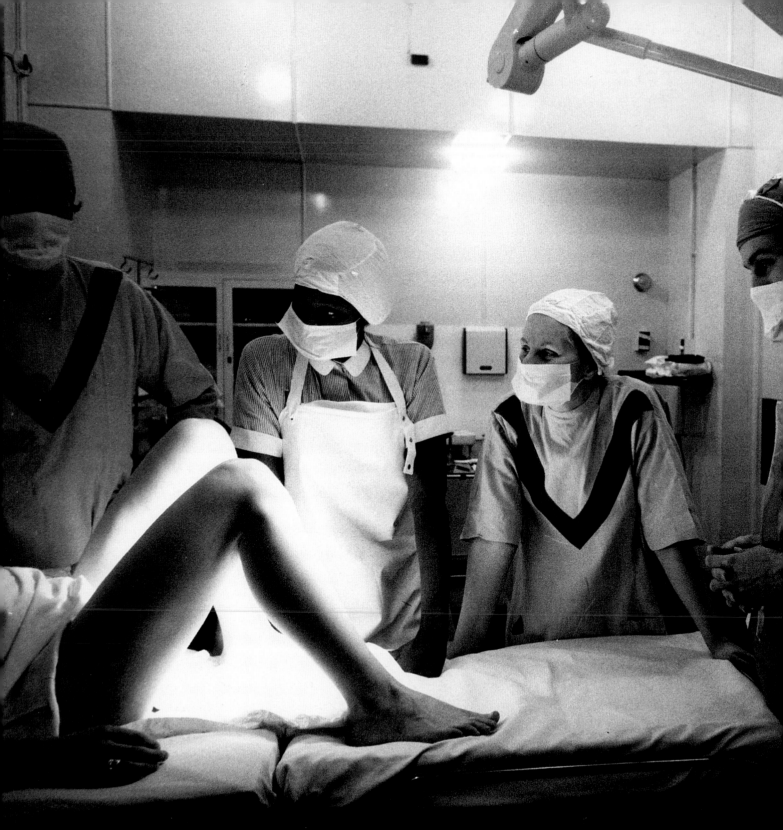

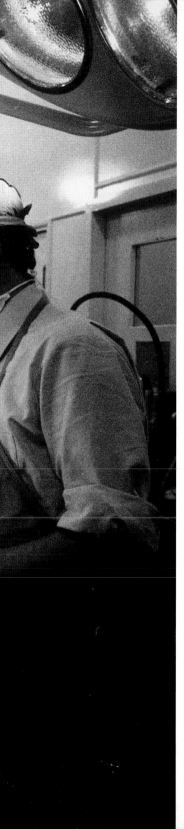

In most hospitals each of these rooms is dominated by a bed surrounded by monitors and other technical equipment. In some university hospitals the bed is replaced by a delivery table with lithotomy stirrups to hold the woman's legs. In the University Hospital in Berlin, the floor, walls and delivery table were all constructed of black rubber. The effect was stark and funereal.

The central position of the bed makes it clear that the woman is supposed to be on it, not moving around, and her posture is restricted and controlled by the professionals managing the labour. Even when the 'three room' model is replaced by a single 'labour/delivery/recovery' room, as it is now in many North American birthing rooms, and increasingly in other hospitals, the bed is still in the middle of the room. The labouring woman can move only with difficulty and within a limited space, and she may not be allowed to get off the bed at all. The motel-like fixtures, the central position of the bed with its bed-side locker, the TV set, the standard chairs, wash basin, the trolley and the resuscitaire dictate the action and determine the interaction of those assisting and observing. The woman is expected to be on the bed and other people position themselves in relation to it. Their relative positions are an expression of the line of command. The senior figure is situated between the woman's legs and others are grouped around him or her at the side of the bed, with the woman's partner, if she has one, in the most subordinate position at the head end, or in countries in which fathers are only just being admitted access to childbirth, sitting in a chair in the corner where he cannot interfere.

Bianca Lepori, an Italian architect who is a specialist in the design of birth rooms that facilitate physiological birth, describes the 'three room' system as providing the 'arrow path', and considers that 'the natural path is a spiral leading towards the centre of a woman's concentration and ability to listen, and therefore towards her own control and choice . . . Women who can give birth naturally do not need particular colours, nor beautiful furniture that reminds them of their homes: They need a space in which to express themselves, in which to wait; they need the space-time to let it happen. The only thing they really need is not to be forced into a particular position. Even pain dissolves with movement; pain killers are a consequence of stillness.'[4]

Left: The relative positions of those in the delivery room are an expression of the line of command.

Shared Knowledge

When simple objects such as a hammock, 'household artefacts . . . which are imbedded in the matrix of daily life', are used in childbirth, the result is 'hands on, collaborative birthing', writes the anthropologist Brigitte Jordan.[5] A Mayan in Yucatan is accustomed to using her hammock to get comfortable. She lies on her back, her side or even her front. Her movement is not restricted and as she feels the baby descending she adjusts her position easily. Her husband, mother, other women in the family and the midwife are equally familiar with hammocks and how they can be used, so they know exactly how to position themselves to give her the best support.

It is quite different for a woman lying on a hospital delivery table. She is no longer held in anyone's arms. The narrowness of the table and the equipment around her prohibit it and mean that there is simply no space for them to get near her. The lower part of her body is draped and isolated from the upper part. She cannot touch it. She cannot see what is happening. And if she has had regional anaesthesia she cannot feel it.

When sophisticated technology is used in childbirth, power is in the hands of those who know how to control and interpret it. Interpreting the squiggles on a print-out from an electronic monitor is often difficult even for those who have been trained to do so. Setting up an intravenous drip, inserting a catheter, giving an epidural, even measuring blood pressure, all require professional skills. The birthing woman turns to her care-givers for information and they turn to the electronic equipment for information. They then decide whether or not to share this with the woman. They may withhold it, telling her not to worry, or give her partial information, or, depending on what they want her to do, give her information which, though inaccurate, is designed to get her to act in a certain way – to push harder or to agree to a Caesarean section, for example, which they consider is in her own and the baby's best interest.

In contrast, when objects are used with which everyone is familiar and which everyone knows how to handle, knowledge is shared. And because knowledge is shared, there is no hierarchy. Though the midwife is respected for her special skills, all the other women present understand birth too, and know how to handle the objects which come in useful in childbirth. Just as women work together in the kitchen or the dairy, so they work together in the birth room. Their activities appear automatic, unspectacular, smoothly co-ordinated. It is as though everyone present knows the steps of the dance and they are all in tune with the same music.

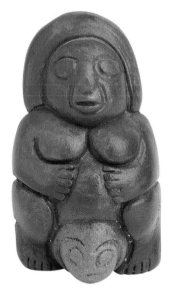

Above and below: Birth sculptures from South America in which the mother is upright.

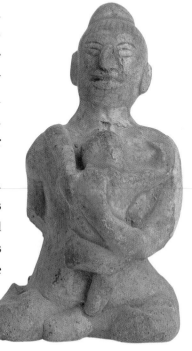

Freedom to Move

The birth room or, in tropical countries, sometimes a clearing in the bush, provides space in which the mother can move, using upright positions in which pain is easier to bear, and spontaneously rock her pelvis to guide the baby down.

In North America women of the Crow tribe gave birth in a special *tepi* made of animal skins, pitched outside the camp. Inside it a fire was burning and soft buffalo skin robes were piled up to make a bed, with two stakes driven into the ground in front of it for the mother to grasp. Until she was ready to push she was encouraged to walk around. A Crow woman, Pretty-shield, tells how the midwife, wearing a buffalo robe and grunting like a buffalo, a sacred beast to the Crow people, told her to 'walk as though you are busy'. To reach the bed she had to walk over four burning coals set between the entrance of the *tepi* and the buffalo skins: 'I had stepped over the second coal when I saw that I should have to run . . . jumped the third coal, and the fourth, knelt down on the robe, took hold of the two stakes, and my first child, Pine-fire, was there with us.'[6]

In the 19th century, a maverick doctor, American George Engelmann[7], and a British medical student, Robert Felkin[8], recorded birth positions in North American native cultures and various African tribes. The descriptions and drawings by these men depict a wide variety of positions and their work remains to this day the most comprehensive analysis of birth postures in the world. If you merely glance at them, the drawings only hint at movement. It is as though a woman adopts a birth posture and gets stuck in it. Yet anthropologists' observations of births in different cultures reveal that this rarely happens. These illustrations showed one, or at most two, segments of what was really movement, and it is this that helps the physiological process of birth and eases pain. The images are like those on a video screen once the pause button has been pressed. In our imagination we need to turn the static image into video and release the action implicit in the posture.

A Plains Indian woman is shown standing with her back to her husband, clasped in his arms. He grasps her firmly so that she can rock, swing her pelvis, bend and straighten her knees, and have the support she needs to move freely in an instinctual response to the power of the contractions.

A woman in Louisiana gives birth while hanging from the branch of a tree, lifting herself off the ground with each contraction. Dr Walter Reed wrote to Engelmann describing how prolonged labour was treated by the Apaches. A rope was tied round the woman's arms and the end thrown over a strong branch above her. Two or three women pulled on the rope until the mother's knees just touched the ground. Another woman knelt beneath her and grasped her round the top of the uterus. During contractions she was suspended from the tree, but also supported and cradled in the woman's arms. From the illustration it is clear that between contractions she was kneeling and with each contraction she

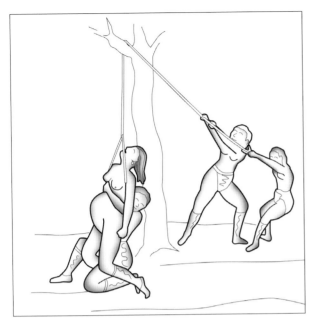

Left: During contractions, an Apache woman is suspended from a tree, while still supported and cradled in the arms of a woman beneath her.

Below: An African woman rests her arms on a log, with smoking herbs burning in a small trench under her perineum.

was hoisted up off the ground, her knees bent and resting on the thigh of the woman beneath her, her toes on the ground. This entailed concerted effort on the part of all four women acting together.

The Sioux woman stood and walked and rocked her pelvis with her arms around the neck of a tall man.[9]

When an African woman is drawn on all fours, with her arms resting on a log placed horizontally on the ground in front of her and with smoking herbs burning in a small trench dug under her perineum, she is actually rolling the log backwards and forwards and rocking her pelvis as she does so. When she stands against a tree holding on to a springy sapling that is hooked between the branches of the tree she is using the sapling to give her support as she rocks her pelvis, alternately bending and straightening her knees, and engaging in a birth dance.

A plaited rope or strip of cloth is often tied to the bedpost or the rafters. Jacqueline Vincent Priya says that when she talked with midwives in northern Thailand they told her that their most important piece of equipment was a rope which they knotted to the house beam. The woman stood holding this, suspending herself by her arms during contractions. Or it might be twisted round her shoulders and under her arms so that it could take her whole weight with each contraction.[10]

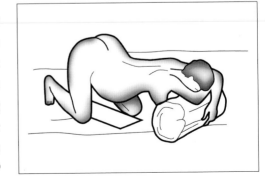

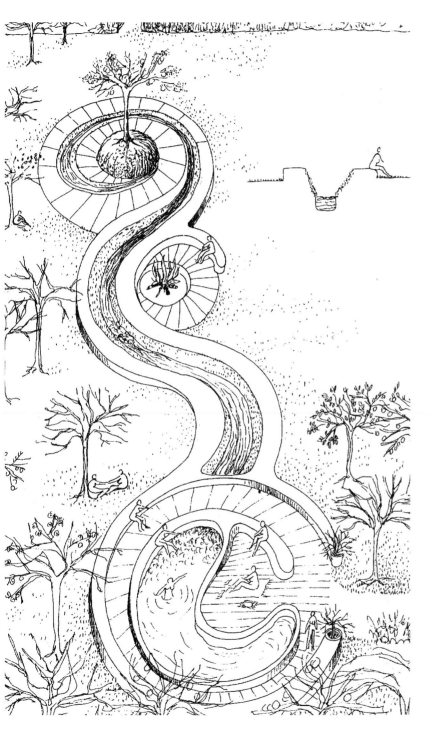

In a hospital in Reykjavik, Iceland, I have seen women labouring using a soft swing hammock hanging from the ceiling in much the same way. The woman leans forward, letting the swing take the weight of her upper body during contractions, or can give her entire weight to it, lifting her feet from the floor and swinging backwards and forwards in much the same way that small children do on playground swings.

Any birth place, wherever it is, serves as a framework for the script of birth. It defines, and often restricts, what can occur within it. If a room is dominated by a high, narrow hospital bed there is little a woman can do but climb on to it. When she is harpooned to electronic equipment movement is still further restricted. Even when the decor is carefully designed to introduce a homely and relaxed atmosphere, in the way the room is laid out, the position of the bed, the chair, the clock, the monitor, the resuscitator and instrument trolley, it is made clear how the woman is expected to behave and where the other participants are to position themselves: the patient here, the birth partner in this chair at her head end, the midwife or doctor there, where a bright lamp shines light on the perineum.

Left: Fanny Di Cara, an Italian architect, imagines a birth garden with flowing water.

Bianca Lepori is an Italian architect who has studied the spontaneous movements women make in labour and how, given an intimate space, they use various parts of it in which to walk, crouch, stand or be on all fours. She designs birth rooms which follow these movements, rather than imposing an expectation that the woman will lie down on the bed or give birth in the centre of the room. She incorporates into her designs a curved birth pool and lighting that can be dimmed, and which is often mysterious and subtle. Another Italian architect, Fanny Di Cara, imagines an open-air garden or courtyard space for birth that includes trees, flowers, flowing water and a log fire.

When women design their own birth space it is very different from the usual hospital delivery room with a large clock and a bed or central delivery table. They choose a pool, candles, soft, indirect lighting, pictures that have special meaning for them, comfortable floor cushions and perhaps a rocking chair and a birth stool. When they are free to move it turns out that they often give birth in a secluded corner of the room.

Birth is movement. A woman who labours at home usually continues with household tasks for as long as she can. She finishes some baking, clears up the kitchen so that it is clean and tidy, fetches washing off the line, gets the children ready for school, sweeps the floor, remakes the bed, perhaps decides to plant out beans that should be in the ground, with the help of her midwife. While she does these things she pauses as each contraction comes, bending her knees slightly and rocking or circling her pelvis.

There is the birth room to prepare so that it is just as she wants it, the children's toys to put away, a bit of ironing to finish. When one of my own labours started I hurried to paint the stairs blue, as the undercoat was just dry. The baby was soon born and when four little girls came into the room to see their new baby sister I noticed that they all had blue toes.

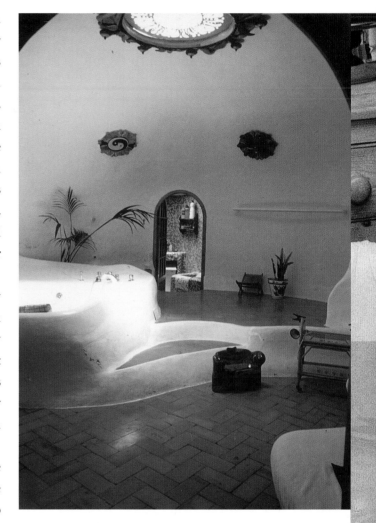

Above: A birth room with a pool. In an environment like this a woman can 'centre down' and respond instinctively to the rhythms of her uterus.

Right: A home birth enables a woman to enjoy the comfort of being in her own, familiar space, with her family around her.

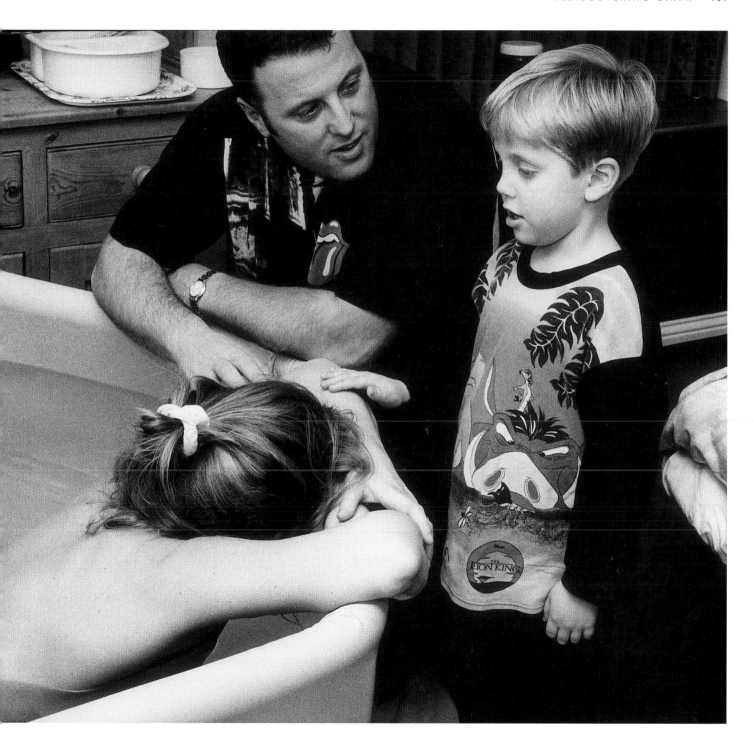

Penny Armstrong, a midwife who has worked with the Amish people in Dutch Pennsylvania, describes her first delivery in an Amish cottage:

Thinking I would find Katie stretched out in her bed, I turned to go up the steps to the back porch. Just then she popped out the back door. She had a paintbrush in her hand.

'Oh,' she said, 'hi . . . Oh, my goodness, I'm not quite ready. I was putting the final coat of lacquer on this rocking chair when I started to have stronger contractions. I just wanted so much for it to be done, so I could rock the baby in it . . .'

She'd cleaned the brush and now she laid it down on some neatly folded newspaper spread out in a corner in the porch. Not only did the rocker look freshly lacquered, but it appeared that the porch floor had been scrubbed and waxed not long ago. She stopped talking for a moment when she stood up, put her hands on her hips, and stretched out her back.

'Is that a contraction?' I asked.

'Yes it is.'

'Is it pretty strong?'

'Yes, I believe it is, and I haven't put that plastic thing on the bed yet.'

We walked through an immaculate kitchen and a spotless living room. She'd gotten her husband off to work, got her toddler up, washed, fed, and dressed, cleaned up the breakfast dishes, straightened up the living room and painted a rocking chair. I think it was about 8:30 in the morning.

Penny examined Katie and found her nine centimetres dilated.

She stopped again for another contraction, and as soon as it passed she went back to spreading out the plastic sheet over the mattress cover. I was supposed to be helping her, but I had trouble concentrating. I kept staring. The woman was nine centimetres dilated and she was bustling about furiously.

We finished making up the bed, then she thought maybe she'd change from her dress into a gown. Next thing I knew, she'd hopped onto the bed. Her face was flushed and she was ready to push.[11]

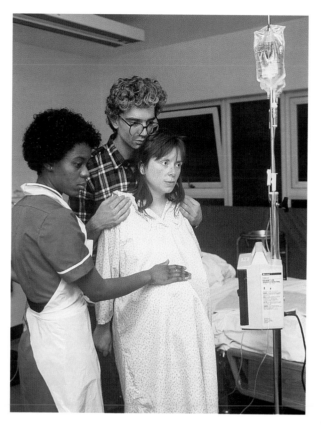

Above: Moving freely in a hospital environment is usually difficult.

At home a woman usually keeps moving. In hospital she is often put to bed. If she wants to move there may be little space unless the bed can be wheeled out of the room or she resorts to walking up and down the corridor. The supine position, with the woman flat on her back, is acknowledged to be dangerous, but it is often easiest to monitor a patient, introduce a catheter and attach her to whatever equipment is being used when she lies like this. Any movement may interfere with the monitor print-out. When a woman lies flat the heavy uterus is tilted down on to the *vena cava*, compresses it and slows the blood flow back through the veins in her legs. This can lead to low blood pressure and oxygen deprivation for the baby as well as herself. It is why, in modern hospitals, women are usually asked to lie on their sides or propped up.

In traditional childbirth other women offer both physical support so that the mother can move without strain, and join in the rhythm of her movements. An American midwife asked a Nicaraguan midwife what she did to help a woman having difficulty coping with her labour: 'She began whimpering, impersonating a woman in distress, and then quickly changing roles, she laughed. "Le invito a bailar" [I invite her to dance], she said.'[12]

A Bedouin Arab girl learns a pelvic dance during the puberty rites that follow her first menstruation and will belly dance to give pleasure to her husband and also when she is in labour. The belly dance is essentially a fertility dance. The night club version for the entertainment of tourists is a distortion of its meaning. The belly dance represents the power of women to produce life.

Women kneel and rock together in the Amazon basin, too. In sculpture and paintings a birth triad constantly recurs: three women in swinging, rocking movement joined in a birth dance, sometimes kneeling or squatting, sometimes sitting, but always moving. This group of three women in close physical contact and moving in unison appears across cultures and through history, in ancient Greece and Rome, in South America and in Africa, and often in midwife-assisted birth today.

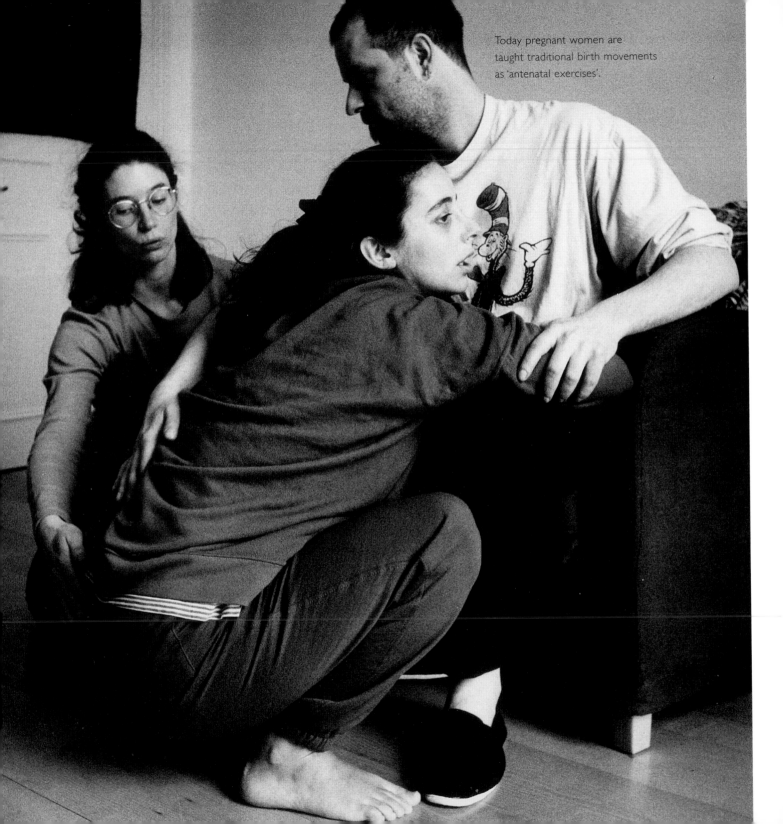

Today pregnant women are taught traditional birth movements as 'antenatal exercises'.

When I interviewed traditional midwives in Fiji, on the tiny island of Vatulele, a crowd of village women gathered to join in the discussion. I was aware that a midwife was struggling to give me the 'correct' answers to my questions, bearing in mind what she knew about hospital birth and the practices of professionally trained midwives. On this island women having first babies are usually transported by air in a very small plane, or by boat, to hospital on the largest island, though some refuse. The traditional midwives often deliver women having second and subsequent babies. This midwife said, 'When the woman lies down . . .' I interrupted her and repeated, 'When she lies down?' and added, 'All over the world women do not usually want to lie down.' The throng of women surrounding us started to laugh, gesticulate and explain, 'No, we don't lie down. We swing along!' and they broke into a vigorous pelvic dance, in which the children clustering round and the midwife and I joined. It was a Fijian birth dance.

In a medicalised birth culture pregnant women are taught these same movements as 'antenatal exercises'. When Janet Balaskas first introduced Active Birth in the 1970s and women started to learn how to move in childbirth it seemed revolutionary. But in reality it was a rediscovery of ways in which women have always given birth. Immobility was imposed on women in the 19th century when doctors wanted their patients to lie flat on their backs so that they could examine them easily. Freedom to move was a return to the roots of women's birth knowledge.

This conflicted with the obstetric management of birth and remains problematic for many doctors who, while they may accept that it helps to reduce pain and is a 'distraction' for their patients, treat it as a concession to women's wishes in the early first stage of labour, which is replaced by oxytocin stimulation of the uterus and an epidural as soon as the patient is beginning to tire, or when dilatation of the cervix does not progress at a normal rate. When a woman is not tethered to machines in labour, a midwife who is sensitively in tune with her birth rhythms often moves with the mother in what is essentially the same birth dance.

There is evidence that activity during childbirth not only relieves pain and reduces emotional stress, but also helps the baby to descend and rotate into the best position for birth.[13] Inactivity, especially when a woman is lying on her back in bed, makes pain more difficult to bear, increases emotional stress and impedes the baby's descent and rotation into the correct position. It also reduces blood flow to the baby, and therefore the oxygen that reaches it from the mother's bloodstream, which is filtered through the placenta.

If a woman is not only in bed but further immobilised because she has had an epidural or is knocked out with opiates (pethidine or meperedine), and is attached to an intravenous drip and electronic equipment that makes movement impossible, labour is not only prolonged, but the normal physiology of birth may be further impeded.

Every nurse and midwife knows that if the electronic monitor indicates that the baby's heart is dipping, the first thing to do is to get the mother to turn on her side or to change position so that she is more upright. Or she may tell the mother to ignore the monitor because it has not been working properly all day, and give it a good kick.

Pelvic movement in childbirth is not an esoteric 'ethnic' practice. Circling, rocking and slanting the pelvis (the latter by lunging or walking up and down stairs) opens up the bony outlet to its widest diameter and guides the ball of the baby's head down in the right direction. If contractions are too weak, something which is more likely to happen if a mother is immobilised and if the pelvis is rigid, this process takes longer, and may never occur at all, resulting in deep transverse arrest of the head as it starts to turn but cannot complete its rotation.

In an environment where a woman gives birth without constraint, embarrassment or feeling that she has to put on a performance, she moves like this spontaneously. Sometimes the movement is slight, hardly noticeable to an observer. But it is often unmistakable. In the same labour a woman may combine minimal and exaggerated movements, depending on what her body is telling her at the time. Though it is often taken for granted that once fully dilated she lies down and stays in position, a woman usually struggles to move her pelvis in the second stage of labour. But this is difficult if she is told sternly, 'Keep your bottom on the table!', if her legs are fixed in lithotomy stirrups, or if she is anaesthetised from the waist down.

Dr Michelle Harrison, whose book describes her residency in obstetrics and gynaecology at a major American hospital, says:

Birth is a creative process, not a surgical procedure. I picture dancers on a stage. Once, doing a pirouette, a woman sustained a cervical fracture as result of a fall; she is not paralysed. We try to make the stage safer, to have the dancers better prepared. But can a dancer wear a collar around her neck, just in case she falls? The presence of the collar will inhibit her free motion. We cannot say to her, 'this will be entirely natural except for the brace on your neck, just in case'.

It cannot be 'as if' it is not there because we know that creative movement and creative expression cannot exist with those constraints. The dancer cannot dance with the brace on. In the same way the birthing woman cannot 'dance' with a brace on. The straps around her abdomen, the wires coming from her vagina, change her birth.[14]

Squatting and Kneeling

Women all over the world spontaneously squat, kneel, stand or lean forward as they give birth. In the 19th century a doctor described how he found a black woman in Georgia, USA, kneeling on a mat with her head and elbows on the seat of a rocking chair and her body almost horizontal. He saw that the baby's head had been born, that it was very large, and that there was shoulder dystocia (that is, the baby was so big that the shoulders were stuck). As each contraction came her body moved backward until her buttocks rested on her heels. In the interval between contractions she glided forward again. In this way she gave birth spontaneously to 'an enormously large child'.[15]

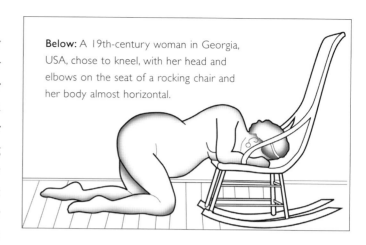

Below: A 19th-century woman in Georgia, USA, chose to kneel, with her head and elbows on the seat of a rocking chair and her body almost horizontal.

This was also how Maori women delivered their babies. The late Dame Whina Cooper, who was born in 1895, described to me how she helped her mother give birth to her sister:

A mother can more or less look after herself. She is trained to look after herself. My mother was giving birth and came into my arms. I went before her and I knelt down and she put her arms round my neck. I was 12 at the time. In hospitals today women are made to lie down. But the Maori women squat or kneel.

In the United States in the 1880s George Engelmann entered into a lively correspondence with other doctors who discussed with him the benefits of squatting. A Dr Campbell in Augusta, Georgia, USA, described how one of his patients had a very long labour in which he decided to use forceps, 'but just then in one of the violent pains, she raised herself up in bed and assumed a squatting position when the most magic effect was produced. It seemed to aid in completing delivery in the most remarkable manner, as the head advanced rapidly, and she soon expelled the child by what appeared to be one prolonged attack of pain. In subsequent parturition, labor appeared extremely painful and retarded in the same manner; I allowed her to take the same position, as I had remembered her former labor, and she was delivered at once, squatting'.[16]

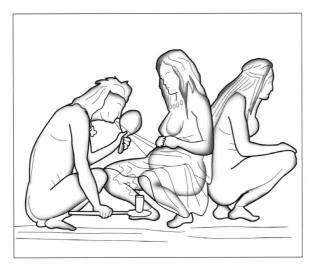

Left: A woman of the Pawnee tribe squats, with another woman squatting back to back with her, and her husband blowing a herbal infusion onto the perineum to help the tissues fan out.

Dr John Williams, a doctor with the Green Bay Indian agency, described how a woman of the Pawnee tribe squatted in childbirth, with another woman squatting back to back with her.[17] Kneeling positions are very common, too. The Blackfoot Sioux woman kneels, leaning forward and grasping a *tepi* pole or heavy staff, with her head resting on her arms. Dr Reamy, a physician in Ohio, wrote:

I have found in my practice ten or twelve different women, who had frequently borne children before, who insisted, with a perseverance and determination that I dared not resist, in being out upon the floor, down upon their knees, leaning backwards so that the buttocks almost touched the heels. The husband knelt behind the wife, with his arms around her, his broad strong hands acting as a pad for the abdomen, and making pressure during pains . . . her shoulders resting against the man's chest. These women insisted that this was the only position in which they could comfortably and successfully be delivered.[18]

Sometimes the woman is in a position in which she is guarding her own perineum. In southern Africa, for example, the woman may kneel, legs wide apart, with her heels supporting her perineum.[19] A woman in central Africa may grasp the branch of a tree which is laid horizontally between two other trees, bending her knees into a squatting position as she pushes. Between contractions she walks slowly up and down. A similar practice is traditional in rural Colombia, where the woman squats holding on to a springy

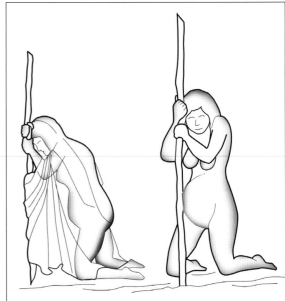

Right: A Blackfoot Sioux woman kneels, leaning forward and grasping a *tepi* pole or heavy staff, with her head resting on her arms.

sapling laid horizontally between two stakes set in the ground. This grasping bar is fixed at the level of her pelvis. Another variation in Africa is a vertical stake that has been driven firmly into the earth. The mother walks round it in a circle until a contraction begins, and then squats down holding it. Or she simply leans against the outside wall of her hut, using it to support her back as she squats down. Sometimes a lump of wood is used as a birth stool. Robert Felkin describes how in one tribe a woman gave birth in a secluded spot near running water. Other women beat tom-toms or blew horns as she squatted on a log and pushed her baby out.[20]

A Brazilian obstetrician, Moyses Paciornik, studied the birth practices of the indigenous people of southern Brazil, the Caingangeery, Choclang and Guarani tribes. He found that after having sometimes very large families, the pelvic floors of tribal women were still in good condition with strong muscles, and that few suffered incontinence or prolapse. But younger women who were delivered by hospital-trained nurses often had the pathological conditions that affect women in modern civilisation: torn muscles, stress incontinence and prolapse. The older women gave birth squatting. The younger women were made to lie supine, told to hold their breath and push as hard as they could, and had episiotomies.

Dr Paciornik decided to change his own practices and asked women to squat or to stand. The result was that women in his care were more likely to have an intact perineum or only a minor tear.[21]

An American study of squatting and pushing in the second stage of labour, compared a randomly selected group of 100 women who squatted and 100 who were in a semi-recumbent position. It revealed that those who squatted – both first-time mothers and those who had had babies previously – had a shorter second stage, the primiparas twenty-three minutes less and the multiparas thirteen minutes less. Those who squatted were much less likely to have oxytocin stimulation in the second stage and had fewer deliveries assisted with forceps or ventouse. They had fewer perineal tears, and if they did have one it was less severe. They also had fewer episiotomies.[22] Other studies bear out the value of getting women up off their backs and into upright or semi-upright positions, and reveal that when a woman squats with support she experiences less birth pain and there is less risk of perineal trauma.[23]

Right: A South American sculpture of birth-giving, with the woman upright and active.

In many cultures a woman squats between her husband's or another woman's thighs, or sits on someone's lap. Maori women used to give birth between the thighs of a grandfather or other spiritually powerful senior man in the tribe, either sitting or standing, leaning back against him and swaying together. In the Andaman Islands the husband sits on the ground with legs outstretched, facing a wall, and the woman sits between his thighs with her knees bent and her feet against the base of the wall so that she can fix herself for pushing.

A similar position was employed well into the 19th century by American women in rural areas. Engelmann remarked that the obstetric chair 'is merely an imitation of the more pliable and sensitive support afforded by the husband or assistant'.[24]

Women in Ohio, Pennsylvania, Missouri, Georgia and the mountains of Virginia, USA, gave birth like this, often using ladder-back chairs as well, one for the husband to sit on and another on its side to give the mother extra support under her thighs. Because these chairs were near the ground, it was simple for a woman to get up and walk about if she wanted to, and then to cuddle up on her husband's lap again. A Dr E. G. Stevens wrote that when he started in practice in Lebanon, Ohio, USA, they used 'two old-fashioned, straight-backed chairs', one upright and the other turned on its side. 'A few old comforters on this framework completed a very comfortable couch, the husband took his seat first, astride, the wife reclining in his arms.' If labour was slow, 'the patient was walked about or assumed any other position as dictated by fancy or impulse; the position of the accoucheur was upon an inverted half bushel measure, so placed that he sat just between the limbs of the patient'. He went on to say, 'This position

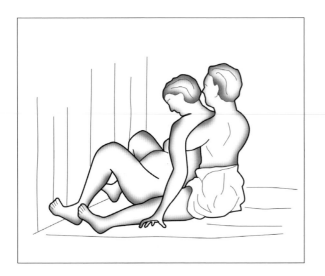

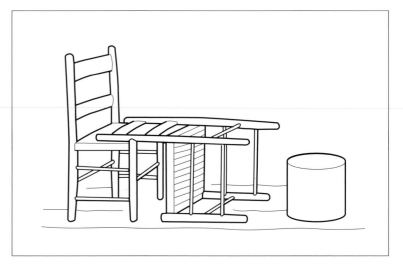

was certainly not a bad one for all parties with the exception of the husband who, in tedious cases, suffered rather severely, but then this little tax on his affectionate nature was, in those days, considered the very least return he could make for the mischief he had occasioned.'[25]

Sometimes three chairs were set in a triangle. The husband sat on one of them with a sheet or towel round his thighs so that it formed a hammock seat for his wife. Two women sat on the chairs opposite to hold the woman's outstretched hands and support her knees, and she placed her feet on the rungs of their chairs.

Birth Stools and Chairs

Birth stools and chairs evolved from lap-sitting and squatting positions. They were low, simple, cut-out wooden shapes that enabled a woman to squat with support. They had no backs to them. The mother was cradled in women's arms and could move her pelvis freely. Among indigenous peoples in South America, stools like this are often still used by traditional midwives.

As time went on, in Europe stools became more elaborate, with low backs to them. This immediately reduced pelvic mobility. But it was convenient because a woman could squat on one without having others supporting her from behind. Engelmann heard of a carpenter in a German village whose wife had such an easy labour while sitting on his lap that he was soon required to attend all the births in the village. 'Finally not a woman in the place would be confined in any other way than on this good man's lap.' He found this such a nuisance that he designed a birth chair.

Far left: In the Andaman Islands the husband sits on the ground with legs outstretched, facing a wall, and the woman sits between his thighs with her knees bent and her feet against the base of the wall.

Left: In Colonial America two old-fashioned straight-backed chairs, one upright and the other turned on its side, formed a birthing couch. The father sat on the chair with the woman between his thighs.

Right: Sometimes, three chairs were set in a triangle.

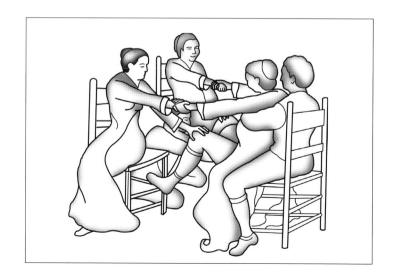

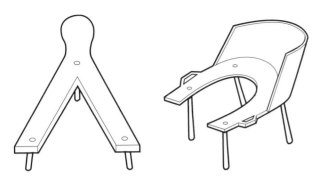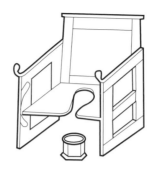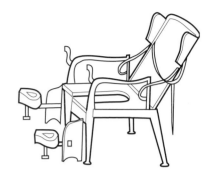

One 16th-century version of a birth stool was a two-seater. The woman could sit on her helper's lap, both of them supported by the stool.

Above: From simple stool to elaborate birth chair.

In wealthier households, especially as doctors took over childbirth, birth stools became increasingly elaborate chairs. At first these were simple structures, but higher off the ground than stools, so that the doctor could sit comfortably in front of the labouring woman and see and feel without the indignity of getting down on the floor.

The chairs became more and more complicated, with footrests, bits that could be lifted off for delivery, sometimes elaborate decoration, and even upholstery. It became harder and harder for a woman to move. She was encased on a kind of rococo commode or birth throne.

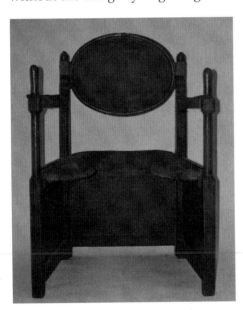

Above: Collapsible birth chair, c. 1700-1830.

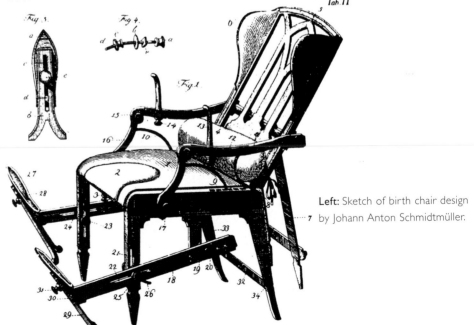

Left: Sketch of birth chair design by Johann Anton Schmidtmüller.

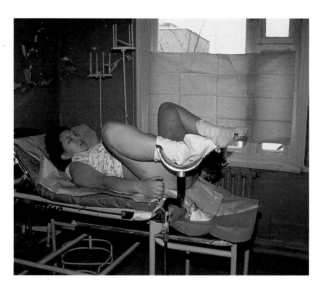

The next development was to tip the woman up on her back on a narrow table and raise her legs. She was held in position with knotted bandages and then, once the 19th-century Industrial Revolution was at its height, with metal restrainers, cuffs and stirrups. In Eastern Europe and the former Soviet Union women still give birth fixed in lithotomy stirrups. A study in St Petersburg reveals that 75 per cent deliver in stirrups, even following a health intervention programme designed to introduce evidence-based care.[26]

With the invention of plastics, delivery chairs and tables could be made relatively light-weight and be easily cleaned and assembled, with the added advantage that the woman could sit up or be speedily tipped on her back, depending on the obstetrician's style of management. In some birth chairs the woman was placed in position with her wrists and ankles held by hand and leg cuffs, and shoulder restrainers were used to prevent her from lifting or moving her head.

Some of these birth chairs are elegantly designed and sinuous as cusped lily petals. They cleverly manage to avoid looking like medical equipment. But the plastic surface is rigid and unyielding and the electronic controls are often out of reach of the woman who is sitting in the chair. Physical support provided by metal and plastic is very different from support by another human body. However well designed, it is less flexible and is unable to respond to subtle messages from the birthing woman – that she wants to shift her weight a little, to change position, or that she seeks pressure against a particular part of her back to ease pain. Compared with any birth chair a companion who holds, clasps, massages and caresses her, and who is sensitive to the physical support she seeks at any particular moment, is superb.

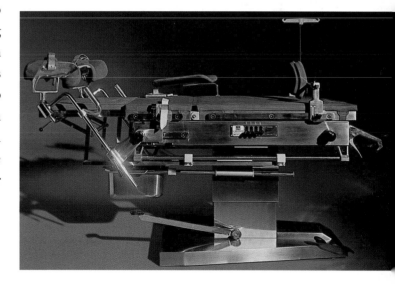

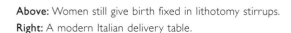

Above: Women still give birth fixed in lithotomy stirrups.
Right: A modern Italian delivery table.

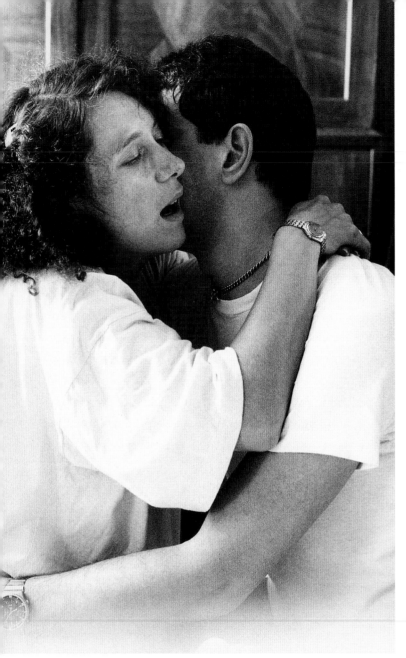
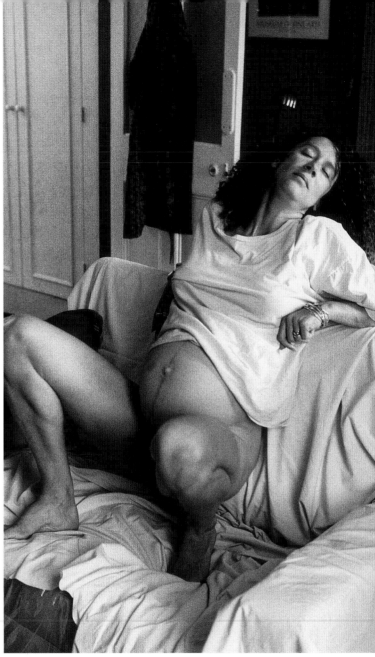

The latest models of birth chairs permit changes in position and allow the lower back to be free. The ideal chair, however, will not only enable a woman to move without constraint, but allow space for a birth companion as well as the mother. For many women, beanbags on the floor or a couple's double bed remain the most comfortable places in which to give birth.

Above: A birth partner who holds, clasps, massages and caresses is better than any mechanical equipment.

Birth Dance in Water

Where water is available, midwives often use it to ease pain in the form of hot compresses and to offer a labouring woman a powerful visual image of the uninterrupted flow of liquid, which can have a strong positive psychological effect. When labour is difficult in peasant Greece, the midwife or the helping women may pour water through the sleeve of the husband's shirt or down the chimney. In Jamaica, the *nana* soaks a cloth in hot water and cocoons the mother within it. English midwives traditionally helped a woman in the first stage of labour into a warm bath, and in diverse cultures immersion in water is used by women as a way of handling menstrual and birth pain.

On some islands in the southern Pacific, women went down to the sea to give birth in the shallows. In New Zealand the women of one Maori tribe in the hills gave birth in a sacred river. But water birth – immersion in a birth pool – is a modern invention. In most societies women have never before had access to large quantities of water and the means of heating it. They have had to carry every drop of water from the well, stand-pipe or river, and must still often walk for miles bearing the family supply. In rural areas of Jamaica in the 1960s, midwives prided themselves on requiring only one large jug of water when attending a woman in labour. Water was a luxury.

When Dr Michel Odent first offered women the chance of labouring in water in his clinic at Pithiviers, he did not plan for them to give birth in water. This happened only because labour progressed quickly once the woman was in the pool and there was no time for her to get out. The first water birth he attended took him so much by surprise that he paddled into the pool in his socks.

Women who experience the benefits of immersion in water often insist on staying in the pool for the birth. Sometimes this is an ordinary household bath. But one problem with a bath is that the sides are often narrow so that the woman cannot move easily. It may also be difficult to make the water deep enough to cover her lower torso. Instead, she is sitting in a puddle. Once birth pools were on the market there were new possibilities, above all of movement in water.

Once floating in a pool, a woman in labour can move unencumbered. The water bears some of her weight and she has the sense of being in her own private world within the margins of her pool. The result is that she moves spontaneously in a way that is common in a wide range of birth cultures. She squats, kneels, lies on her side, goes on to all fours, or crouches forward holding on to the side of the pool. She may rest with her head and shoulders supported by the pool edge and let her body float, or lie forward with elbows and head on the edge. She may also explore gliding movements, using her arms to glide forwards and backwards during contractions or to turn from her back to one side, or from one side to the other, rolling her pelvis over as she does so. She lunges, bending one or both knees and pushing away from the side of the pool. She rolls her knees from side to side so that she is also rolling her pelvis. In water these instinctive movements come quite naturally. She rediscovers birth postures and movements that are common to traditional birth cultures all over the world.

The irony is that just when research in northern industrialised cultures has revealed the advantages of mobility during labour, immersion in water, and upright and semi-upright positions for birth, and as ways are being explored of achieving this in the context of the medical model for birth, by offering mobile epidurals and having birth chairs which allow an upright position, for example, traditional birth attendants throughout Africa, South America, the Far East and Oceania are being taught to change their age-old birth practices and insist that the mother is in a supine position.

In Guatemala, for example, midwives sometimes refuse to attend a woman who is not lying down. In their training courses they have been led to believe that squatting is dangerous, because the baby could hurt its head on the ground, with resulting brain damage.[27] In India, *dais* are being trained to make the mother lie down instead of giving birth on a soft bed of warm sand which can be easily swept up afterwards. Government health authorities and international agencies provide plastic sheets at 50 rupees a time. The plastic tears, to save money it gets reused for the next patient, or the *dai* decides to use old fertiliser bags instead. It would be safer, and more comfortable for the mother, if they returned to the custom of using sand.

All human cultures are remarkably adaptive, inventing ways of confronting a hostile environment, extreme climactic conditions and inadequate resources. When education is all one way, when trainers coming from within a medical model of childbirth communicate their beliefs and methods to personnel in developing countries without any corresponding learning from indigenous cultures, we are impoverished.

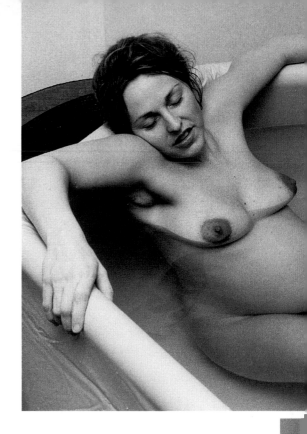

Above and right: In water a woman in labour can move unencumbered, and she rediscovers movements that are common to traditional birth cultures all over the world.

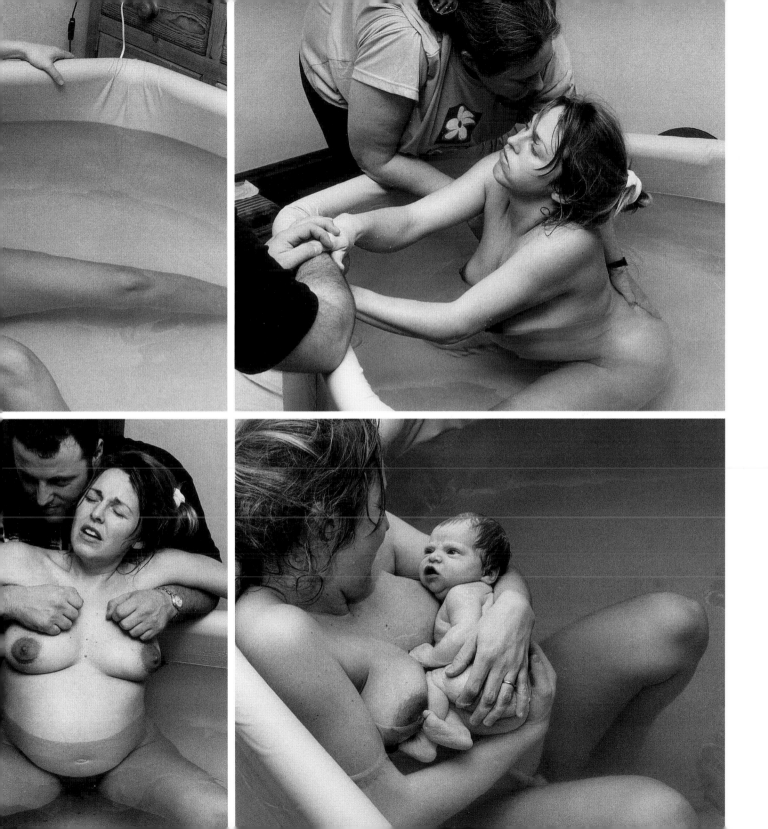

Chapter 7

Birth and Touch

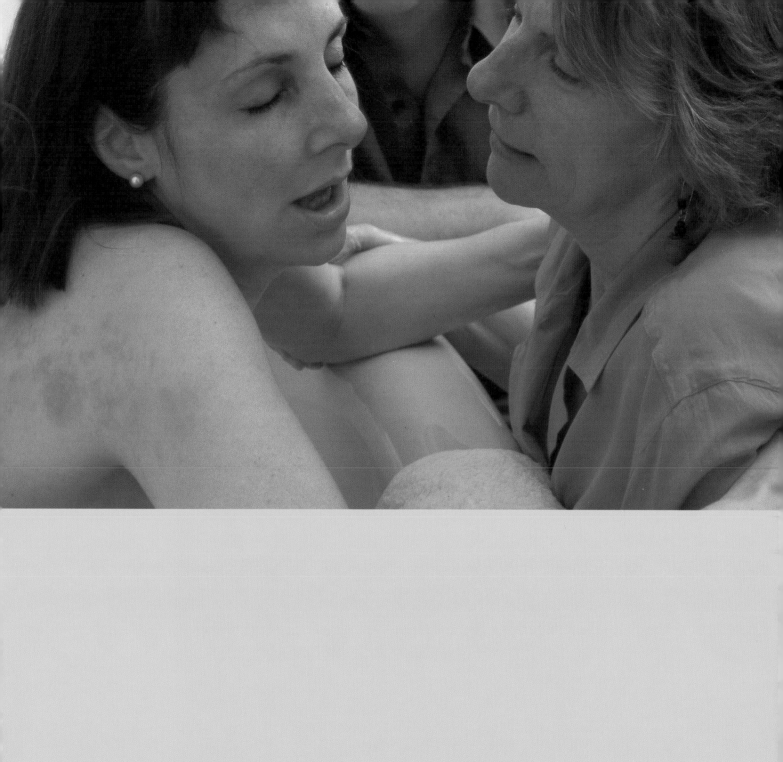

A vital element in both the art and the science of midwifery is the skill of the midwife's hands. Together with her eyes and her ears, her hands are her most valuable tool, transforming the potentially pathological into the normal. But they are more than a tool. She communicates with them. She receives information through the sensitivity of her touch, and gives comfort, confidence and courage by touch. A good midwife knows exactly how and when to touch, just as she also knows when to be hands off.

Northern industrialised culture places great emphasis on verbal communication. But anyone who journeys south to Mediterranean cultures will notice that people communicate more by gesture, whole body movements and touch. The anthropologist Margaret Mead once remarked that when she was lecturing in South America the members of her audience were in such close physical contact that with just two electrical charges she could have electrocuted the lot of them. Whatever this suggests about her attitude to the audience, it reveals that people come closer, reach out, stroke, embrace, and cling more readily in southern countries than in Northern Europe and America. The word 'midwife' is Old English for someone who is 'with' a woman: not just comforting, not just near, but in contact. Modern obstetrics is part of a 'no touch' – or at least 'touch gingerly' – culture. The idea of midwifery as part of a 'touch' culture does not fit comfortably with the medical model of birth.

Touch can only be understood within its social context. Each culture has a language of touch in childbirth. An Orthodox Jew may not touch his wife once she has had a 'show' or her membranes have ruptured, because she is unclean. Even mopping her brow with a cold cloth would risk physical contact, so is prohibited. While couples in Orthodox families in British cities accept this rule with equanimity and acknowledge it as an important part of their cultural identity, young Jewish migrants newly arrived from Israel find it a difficult precept to obey, since within Israel such regulations have become more relaxed over the years.

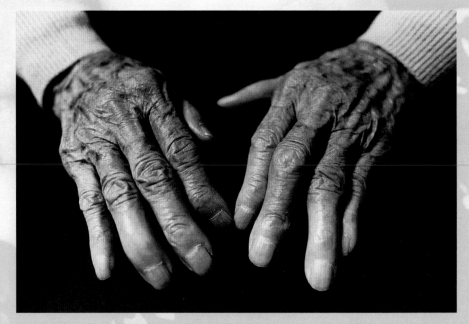

A vital element in midwifery is the skill of the midwife's hands.

An elderly Chinese woman told me that when she gave birth at home some sixty years ago, the local midwife held her hand and 'when she felt the pulsating of my fingers she knew the birth door was opening and the baby is going to go out'. Yet contemporary studies of Chinese women giving birth in hospital reveal that they do not want midwives or other health professionals to touch them in labour unless absolutely necessary. They appreciate verbal praise. Close physical contact by strangers is considered rude and offensive and they wish to control levels of intimacy with everyone who is not part of the close family relationship. To touch uninvited is to invade their privacy.[1] Yet when women gave birth at home, the midwife was already a friend of the family and her touch was welcomed; it is the move from home to hospital that has produced a distance in the relationship between a woman and her midwife and made touch threatening.

At the other extreme, an American midwife describing a birth in Nicaragua said, 'There was no moment during the labor when the midwife's hands were not touching the young woman giving birth – hands touching to receive information and touching to give encouragement.'[2]

Throughout Malaysia the traditional midwife's training is based on touch. The *bidan kampung* learns by placing her hands over a pregnant woman's uterus and discovering the fetal parts. She observes her teacher manually adjusting the position of a fetus which is misaligned, and performing external rotation from breech to cephalic (head down) presentation. She rests her hands over her teacher's to develop tactile understanding of exactly how to perform these manoeuvres. She learns how to massage with coconut oil and with a ritually 'hot' paste during and after the birth, how to diagnose the strength of contractions by touch, and to feel the mother's pulse, since labour is not considered to be progressing well until the pulse beats slightly faster than normal. She introduces her finger into the vagina to judge the descent of the baby's head, and if there is delay once the baby's head crowns, she massages the mother's head with coconut oil, lifts some strands of hair over the face where the mother's fontanelle would have been at her own birth, and recites, 'If this hair is slippery, you will slip out; if this hair is not slippery, you will not slip out.' She ties touch to suggestion, a combination that can have a powerful psychosomatic effect. Once the baby is born she massages its arms and legs and binds the child in swaddling cloth. Then she bathes the mother in warm water to which 'hot', scented leaves have been added, and gives her a massage. The Malaysian midwife learns through touch and her practice is based on touch combined with ritual.[3]

Touch may be warmly welcomed and looked forward to as a normal part of care in childbirth or it may be culturally insensitive and personally intrusive. In a technocratic culture, where a medical model strictly defines the purpose of and justification for touch, women reporting traumatic birth experiences often describe touch which they perceived as assault: 'When she tried to dilate my cervix manually it was terribly painful'; 'They touched me so roughly I felt just like a piece of meat.'

During the 17th and 18th centuries, touch and the ability to learn from touch what was happening to the fetus and to the woman's body formed the essence of obstetrics. This was because a male doctor was not allowed to look at his female patient's genitals. When a male midwife or 'accoucheur' was called in he would have a sheet tied around his neck like a huge bib, rather like the kind that diners in a fish restaurant may wear when eating lobster. It extended over the patient's body, and he had to fumble beneath the sheet and feel his way into her vagina and up to the cervix and the presenting part, while watched by a crowd of women helpers. It was all done by touch.

By the 19th century the bib sheet had disappeared, but the doctor's expertise was still assessed almost entirely by his diagnostic skill derived from what was called 'The Touch'. Everything he did, including vaginal examinations, first had to be negotiated with the women attending, who observed him with critical eyes and strong disapproval of male involvement in childbirth. If he did not have 'The Touch' no amount of book-learning or other abilities could make up for its absence. The discretion, grace and reassurance with which doctors employed touch separated the bumblers from those with acknowledged flair. In the best hands, touch had the quality of magic. Letters in medical journals of the time discussed

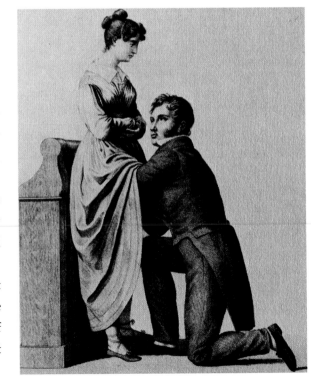

how, when and with what etiquette and manner of bearing a doctor should make a vaginal examination, and there was lively debate as to whether the doctor should stare into the patient's eyes or gaze into the far corner of the room so that she could be quite sure that he was not looking at her genitals. One solution was to have the woman standing, fully dressed, while the doctor knelt on one knee in front of her and slipped a hand beneath her long skirts and into her vagina. Knickers had an open crotch, so a woman could urinate standing up without removing any clothing. This made the doctor's task easier than it might have been if he had had to find his way past her lower garments as well. Yet only the fingers of an experienced and competent man could travel between her petticoats direct to the goal with assurance.[4]

By the dawn of the 20th century it was taken for granted that examination of the vagina and manipulation of the fetus were essential obstetric skills, but discussion about the conduct of touch had evaporated. In fact, medical texts of the time omit reference to touch almost entirely.

Joseph DeLee, who oversaw the birth of modern obstetrics in the United States, devotes six pages of his book, *Obstetrics for Nurses,* to asepsis during labour, and just one paragraph on how to handle the labouring woman. Writing about the second stage, he says:

If the patient, as is often the case, wishes to hold a human hand, have the husband prepare his hands and put on a sterile gown. He may thus help in the labor close up. The patient may feel better if pressure is made on the small of her back or if that part be briskly rubbed, which the nurse may do. Occasionally washing the hands and face with cold water is also grateful. If the patient should have cramp in her leg, which not seldom happens, the nurse stretches the limb out forcibly and pulls the foot toward the knees.[5]

Throughout the book illustrations show the nurse holding the patient in position for the obstetrician. In the preface he thanks the nurses who conducted these demonstrations, but omits to thank the mothers.

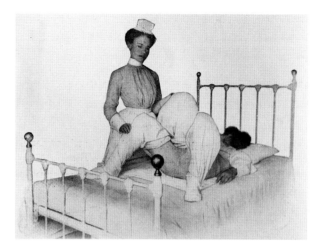

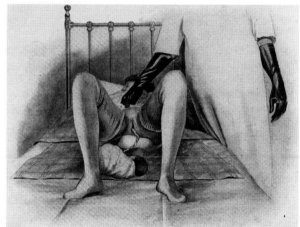

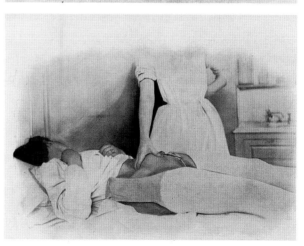

Left: Only the fingers of an experienced and competent man could travel between a woman's petticoats direct to the goal with assurance.

Right: In Joseph DeLee's book illustrations show how the nurse should hold the patient in position for the obstetrician and press firmly on the fundus after delivery.

Touch often conveys messages that conflict with those that are spoken; messages of which the donor may be unaware. At other times touch reinforces the spoken message. It has its own often intricate language; it is not merely a mish-mash of arbitrary signals. And, like spoken language, it can be analysed to try to understand social relationships.

The messages that care-givers convey through touch may come as a complete surprise to them. They did not mean it that way. The ceremonial processes of the labour ward and delivery suite blur the edges of the meanings important in touch. When hospital staff are asked about how they touch, they often deny what they do, or question the reality of what has been observed. Videotape of the behaviour of nurses and doctors in an American hospital during the second stage of labour shows a nurse raising her gloved hand, making a fist with it, and saying, 'You'll feel me touching you, sweetie.'[6] She then pushes her fingers into the woman's vagina and up into her cervix. The signal of the clenched fist raised in the woman's line of sight is one of attack, though her words contradict this interpretation. The hand is held inside the body through two contractions, during which the woman writhes in pain. Obstetrician and epidemiologist Murray Enkin commented on this in a paper entitled 'Do I Do That? Do I Really Do That? Like That?'[7] Reviewing the research he wrote, 'Repeated vaginal examinations are an intrusive intervention of as yet no proved value.'

The medical model of birth restricts touch to certain individuals who have the authority to handle the parturient woman's body and to touch it in clearly defined ways in order to investigate, diagnose, manipulate, control and restrain. Certain parts of the body are out of bounds to everyone but these individuals. When the mother's body is draped in a sterile cloth, even she is not allowed to touch herself below the waist. Her partner may be allowed to mop her brow, kiss her, hold her hand and rub her back, but is not expected to massage her perineum, introduce a finger into her vagina, or touch the baby's head as it is being born. Moreover, when professional care-givers indicate that they are about to set up an epidural, take blood pressure, introduce an intravenous drip or urinary catheter, or put an electrode on the baby's head, the partner is expected to withdraw. In a hospital setting, each participant – the obstetrician, the partner, the nurse or midwife – has rights over a defined territory of the woman's body and is allowed specific kinds of touch.

In the United States a nurse touches a patient to examine, position, restrain and comfort her. But she is not permitted to make the definitive vaginal examination which confirms that the cervix is fully dilated. It is the obstetrician who must do this, and who then says, 'Push!' or 'Do not push!' Nor is the nurse allowed to deliver the baby, except in emergencies. She can catch it if it comes before the obstetrician can get there, but should not usually guard the perineum or control the delivery of the baby's head.[8] I have observed that even a trained midwife in some northern Italian hospitals may not be

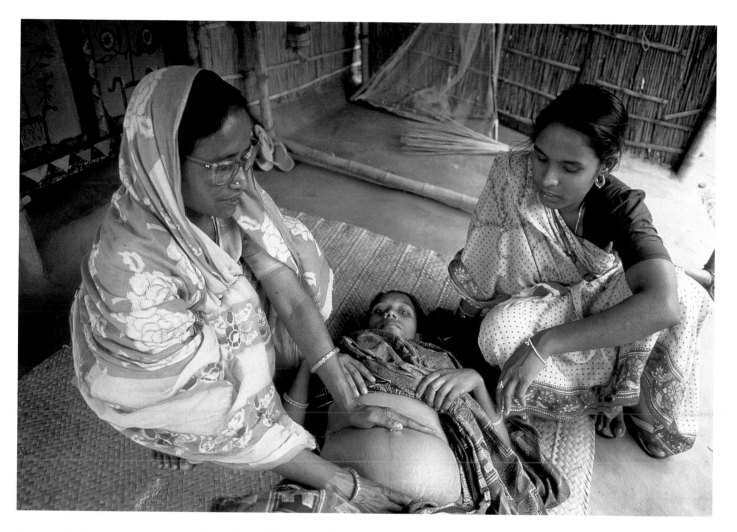

Above: A *dai* abdominally palpates a Bangladeshi woman.

allowed to deliver a baby. That is the prerogative of the obstetrician.

Diagnostic touch is the kind most commonly employed in the medical model of birth. It is often conducted through the agency of an instrument: a blood pressure gauge, the electrode of a fetal monitor, or the clip on the fetal scalp to measure blood gases, for example. The hands are used as a device for measuring or, more often nowadays, to hold an electronic instrument that will make the measurement.

The primary example of diagnostic touch is the vaginal examination. The normal protocol is that this should be performed every two hours throughout labour and every ten minutes in the second stage, with extra examinations if labour does not conform to the norm and dilatation is not progressing at a rate of 1cm every hour. Further vaginal examinations are performed by student doctors and midwives who are learning to perform them.

The vaginal examination has always introduced the risk of infection. In the 19th century this risk was extremely high. In the University Hospital in Budapest, Semmelweis met with huge opposition when he claimed that 'Puerperal fever is caused by conveyance to the pregnant woman of putrid articles derived from living organisms, through the agency of the examining fingers.'[9] But it was true. Medical students performed vaginal examinations without washing their hands between patients, and often after doing autopsies. Rates of puerperal fever on their wards were more than four times higher than on wards where women were attended by midwives.

There is a risk of infection even when examinations are done under sterile conditions in modern hospitals, and the longer the labour the greater the risk, not just because of the length of labour, but because of the greater number of vaginal examinations.[10]

Diagnostic touch also plays an important part in traditional childbirth. Starting as soon as a woman has missed her first period, the Indian *dai* palpates her abdomen to feel the life energy (*jee* or *jeevan*) in her body, and continues to do this regularly through to postpartum. The Colombian *comadro* visits the expectant mother every month to massage her, using oil or lard for lubrication, both to treat backache and in the last six weeks or so to check the baby's position. She uses external version to reposition the baby if she considers it necessary. After doing this she wraps the mother tightly in a binder to maintain an anterior vertex presentation.

The Mexican midwife assesses the height of the fundus of the uterus, palpates the abdomen to discover how the baby is lying, and listens with her ear directly against the mother's abdomen. There are few tools for measurement. The midwife's own eyes, ears and hands make the diagnosis. A doctor described how he called a *partera* (traditional Mexican midwife) to his office to show her how to use a stethoscope so that she could listen to the baby's heart. 'I don't need that,' she said, and handed it back to him. Then she moved her hand across the woman's abdomen. 'Put your instrument here and listen to the heart', she told him 'the heartbeat is here.'[11]

Touch may be both diagnostic and *manipulative,* and these two functions often overlap. A midwife's hands are her most important tool for turning the baby into the correct position for birth. Among the Zapotec of Oaxaca in south-west Mexico, midwives use abdominal massage, *sobada,* and pelvic rocking, *manteada* (literally 'sifting'), to ensure that the baby is in the right position. These skills date back to preColombian times and are effective in turning a baby from posterior to anterior.[12]

A Zapotec *partera* will massage the woman's legs to diagnose tension. By becoming aware of tension in her legs she discovers where the baby is pressing against the woman's spine and causing backache,

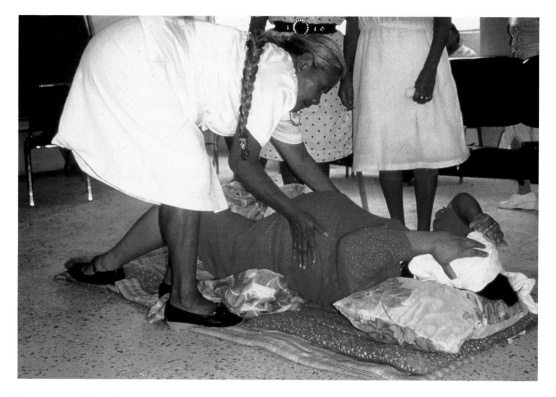

Right: A Mexican *partera* shows how to give the *sobada* rocking massage, an important element in Mayan pregnancy care.

and this shows how the baby should be repositioned. She starts doing this at thirty-two weeks and massage sessions are arranged every fifteen days. As well as massage of the legs, she palpates the abdomen, kneads it, lightly massages it with the sides of her hands, and 'lifts' the baby if the mother has uncomfortable pressure against her bladder and pelvic floor. She massages the woman's back, exerts pressure on the sacro-iliac points, slaps the mother's heels and manipulates her head and neck. About three weeks before the baby is due she may do abdominal massage to 'separate' the baby so that it descends more easily, and give back massage to transmit energy and heat and overcome the 'coldness' which is considered dangerous in pregnancy.

If the baby does need repositioning she asks the woman to lie on her back on the ground, with her knees drawn up and heels flat. Then she places a long shawl, the *rebozo*, under her back and pulls it up at either side so that it cradles her hips. She pulls alternately with her hands to rock the woman's pelvis from side to side in the sling formed by the *rebozo*. She may also do this in the second stage of labour with the woman in a standing position, leaning back against her, to help her to push the baby out. These complex techniques of massage and rocking are now being reassessed and incorporated into modern midwifery skills in Mexico.[13]

An aboriginal tribe in Japan, the Ainu, also used massage to turn the baby from posterior to anterior.[14] Indeed, evidence from many cultures suggests that this is a midwifery practice that has been largely forgotten today.

In the past in Europe and North America, obstetricians often used to turn a baby from breech to vertex in order to avoid Caesarean sections and difficult vaginal deliveries. But over the last twenty years or so, few have learned how to do it and many now consider it not worth the bother. Yet randomised controlled trials have revealed that two out of three babies can be turned, and will stay head down for birth, if rotation is performed after thirty-seven weeks or early in labour. This halves the Caesarean rate for breech births.[15] Modern midwives are not taught how to do this. Nor do they know how to rock and massage babies from posterior to anterior so that the head is in a more favourable position to pass through the cervix and birth canal. Only in countries where professional and traditional midwives have an opportunity to share their skills is this still possible.

In many traditional cultures it is believed that the baby can 'come up' and choke the mother during childbirth. Pressure over the fundus by hand or with a belt or shawl is used to help the baby go down. An Apache midwife will stand behind a woman with her arms around her crossing over her fundus, and with each contraction presses with her hands moving down over the uterus.[16] In my own field research in Jamaica women often talked about the dangers of the baby 'coming up' and choking the mother, and what their midwives did to help avoid it. They kept the baby moving down by massaging its buttocks through the mother's abdominal wall, using pressure over the fundus, and by ensuring that a string or cloth was tied at the level of the fundus not only during labour, but also in pregnancy. Women in both North and South America used what was described by 19th-century observers as a 'squaw belt': a strip of cloth, the ends of which were crossed behind and grasped by the mother, who pulled on it in the intervals between contractions to maintain firm pressure at the top of the uterus.

The idea that the uterus can move out of place and even break from its moorings is an ancient one. The Greeks believed that hysteria was caused by this. *Hustera* is the Greek word for

Right: A Mexican sculpture showing the mother pulling on the *rebozo* around her fundus during a contraction.

uterus. Throughout Europe and North America in the 19th century doctors thought that only a woman could become hysterical because only she had a uterus, and hysteria was a consequence of malfunction of this organ.

In some traditional cultures understanding about the baby's development and its position in the uterus is not specialist knowledge. Instead, it is shared. Maori women used to watch each pregnancy very carefully and assess as a group the condition of the mother and the baby by direct observation. They would then sing about the progress of the pregnancy. If the baby was not growing well or there were any other problems they sang about this, too. No one in the *marae*, the community and religious centre that embodies the identity of the tribe, remained ignorant about what was happening, and nothing was hidden from the mother herself. There is a vast difference between specialist knowledge that is part of the mystique and power of medicine, and knowledge which is shared in this way. Where knowledge is shared, touch is not restricted to certain specialised individuals. As we saw in Chapter 6, birth becomes a dance in which everyone present is likely to take part. In some cultures, indeed, music is played, too.

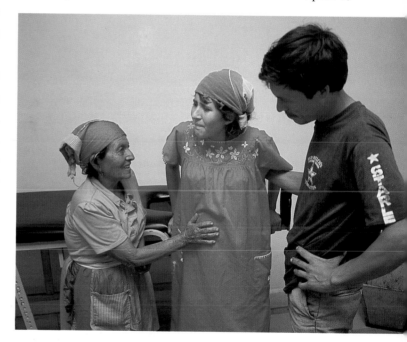

It is not only hands that touch. Helpers use other parts of their bodies too. In both East and West Africa the midwife often uses a foot to provide firm pressure. In Sierra Leone, among the Kaguru of East Africa, the midwife sits facing the mother and supports her perineum with her big toe as the baby's head descends.[17] In India the midwife may use her foot to guard the perineum, and in the first stage presses her heels against the mother's lower back to relieve sacro-lumbar pain.

Much of the touch involved in birth is *comfort* touch. It aims to ease pain and convey a message of sympathy and understanding. At its simplest, comfort through contact is provided via a hand to hold, a shoulder to lean on, or firm pressure in the right place on an aching back. But the hands-on comfort skills of experienced midwives and other female birth attendants go far beyond this.

Above: A traditional midwife in Honduras assesses the strength of a contraction.

We have seen already that the traditional Japanese word for midwife is *samba*, 'the elderly woman who massages'. The heart of traditional Japanese midwifery lies in the use of touch to reposition the baby, to help the woman relax and so let her body work, and to give comfort.

A Mexican *partera* explained that an important part of her work was touching 'as soft as I can'.[18] Yet it is not only the *partera* who touches. The *tendera*, another woman who nurtures the mother during childbirth, also holds and touches. While the *tendera* supports her from behind, the *partera* sits in front of her.

A lubricant oil, cream or lotion is often used, and depending on the culture and the availability of different lubricants this may be animal or vegetable fat, or even juice or vegetable sap. In Micronesia the massage oil is made from coconut cream mixed with finely grated ginger.[19] A midwifery book published in England in the 16th century tells the midwife to 'anoint her hands with the oil of white lilies' and then stroke 'gently with her hands her belly about the naval'.[20] The 1797 edition of the *Encyclopaedia Britannica* advised 'pomatum' (hair oil), butter or warm oil.[21] The idea behind this kind of massage was that oiling and stroking the woman's perineum was not only comforting but enabled the tissues to fan out so that they did not tear as the baby's head and shoulders were born.

In their *Book of Household Management*, published in England in the 18th century, Grace Acton and Letitia Owen recommended pork fat to soften the perineum.[22] And a Victorian book of advice – an odd mix of Aristotle and marriage guidance – counsels the midwife to 'massage the woman's privities with emollient oil, hog's grease and fresh butter.'[23]

Few midwives in modern hospitals massage the woman's perineum. Midwives in independent practice are much more likely to do so, having learned it during their apprenticeship to another midwife. It does not form a part of conventional midwifery education. The practice of using vapour on the perineum is rarer still. Instead, midwives learn how to guard the perineum with a hand as the baby's head descends and bulges it out, and then perform an episiotomy if the tissues become thin and shiny and are under strain. If the woman is having her first baby or the head seems large they may do an episiotomy even without further indications.

Yet comfort touch is not only a question of massage. We have seen already that in preindustrial cultures birth usually takes place within a circle of women who are physically close to the mother and to each other. A British midwife who observed a birth in a village in the Yemen described how the women present stroked, embraced and kissed the mother. 'She was never at a loss of a shoulder to grip, a chest to lean against, or a strong hand to steady an ankle or a knee. If one woman tired or had to return to her children another would quickly take her place.'[24] The anthropologist Brigitte Jordan tells how women help at a Mexican birth: 'With the head helper behind her, not only holding her but physically matching every contraction, the laboring woman is surrounded by intense urging in the touch, sound, and sight of those close to her.'[25]

In many traditional societies, as each contraction starts the whole group of women stirs, and their watching, waiting or casual conversation changes to a wave of focused activity to help her. They support her head, stroke her brow, hold her shoulders or the sides of her abdomen, press on the fundus, press with their knees against the small of her back to ease low backache, and rock or rotate her pelvis.

Comfort touch of this kind is closely linked with *physically supportive* touch, the firm holding that enables a woman to stand, squat or kneel, confident that she has support. It is much easier to move when she has another human body to hold or lean against, or when she is grasped in strong arms by a helper who responds at the onset of each contraction and offers a solid base for whatever position she wants to be in and whatever movement she makes. An 18th-century book, *System of Midwifery*, says that in the Highlands of Scotland a woman in labour usually stands in front of a woman who is taller than herself with her arms around her neck, and the helper supports her back and presses her knees against the mother's knees.[26] The Sioux woman would stand with her arms around the neck of a tall man, and a 19th-century American obstetrician commented, 'I am informed upon credible authority that the young bachelor bucks are most frequently chosen for this service.'[27]

Lap-sitting is another way in which a woman is given solid support. In the past this was common practice in Italy, Germany, Russia, Britain, India, Africa, Peru, the United States and among the Maori. It is a position that is now being rediscovered in modern hospitals.

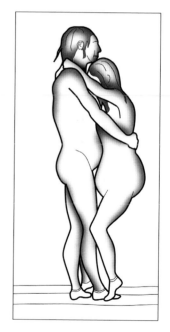

Above: A Sioux woman stands with her arms round the neck of a tall man, his hands pressing in the small of her back.

> **As each contraction starts the whole group of women stirs, and their watching, waiting or casual conversation changes to a wave of focused activity to help her.**

There is another kind of touch, the *blessing* touch. This gives more than comfort – it communicates spiritual power. It may be the power of the ancestors or gods, or that of a supreme spiritual being, or may give a more generalised message of harmony and rightness.

The laying on of hands is one form of blessing touch that summons the Goddess of Birth, or calls on companies of angels. A Jamaican *nana* calls the oil massage she gives an 'anointing'. It has religious connotations. Among the Maori a woman used to give birth sitting between the thighs of her maternal grandfather or mother's brother, or kneel with her head in his lap, as she pushed the baby out on to a sheepskin or carpet of soft leaves. This close physical contact with her grandfather linked her symbolically with the tribal source of spiritual power and conferred *mana*. In Thailand, holy water is sprinkled on the mother's body and the midwife uses this fluid for massage, while in the northern part of the country a sacred formula is pronounced while firmly holding the mother's head and pressing downwards.[28] These are all forms of blessing touch.

The midwife's touch may confer what is perhaps best described as primal energy. In the words of a Mexican midwife, 'The hands of the midwife serve as a medium to give the woman new contraction force.' This particular midwife rests one hand on the woman's uterus while raising the other towards the heavens and asks the sun, moon and God to give the mother fresh energy.[29]

The study of *therapeutic* touch is now incorporated into nursing degree programmes in many American universities. This is quite different from massage to release tension in muscles. An American nurse, Dolores Krieger, was the first person to use this term in a nursing context and she states that it is not associated with any religion or belief, but, she suggests, works through electron resonance.[30]

Restraining touch may be used in childbirth, too. This is common in large, inner city hospitals in North and South America and other countries in which women who cannot afford private care are herded into hospitals where over-worked and highly stressed staff concentrate on crowd control. They try to keep work flowing smoothly, while dealing with women from different ethnic and often deprived backgrounds, who may not speak or understand the dominant language. In an attempt to manage them, hospital staff summon, guide and give directions by physical contact, placing limbs where they want them, pulling, pushing and restricting movements.

Under these circumstances restraining touch quickly turns into *punitive* touch. A woman's hand is slapped as she reaches to contaminate the obstetrician's 'sterile area'. She is slow to turn into the correct position, and a nurse taps her bottom. During the 1960s I spent some time working in the Victoria Jubilee Hospital in Kingston, Jamaica. There were only two pillows on the delivery wards. They were used to press against the faces of women who were screaming. At that time Jamaica had only just started training midwives in the University Hospital at Mona. All senior midwifery staff had been trained

> **'The hands of the midwife serve as a medium to give the woman new contraction force.'**

abroad, in Britain, or sometimes Canada, and there was a cultural divide between these professionals and the women giving birth in the Jubilee Hospital that catered for the poorest Jamaicans. After watching me climb on to a delivery table to cradle a woman in my arms as she pushed her baby out, a senior midwife asked, 'How can you be interested in them? They are just animals!'

In any hospital where there is marked social distance between care-givers and mothers, and any institution in which authoritarian power is exercised, women giving birth may be anxious that they will be punished if they do not conform. In Britain women sometimes describe lengthy vaginal examinations and manual stretching of the cervix which they perceived as being punishment because they failed to conform to the standard of a 'good patient'. Similarly, when a woman has stated that she does not want an episiotomy but has one anyway, she may interpret this as a punishment because she submitted a birth plan. Care-givers may protest that this is 'all in her mind'. Maybe. But it indicates the powerlessness felt by many women in childbirth.

Some women use the language of rape when they describe how they were touched. They feel 'victimised', 'invaded', 'violated' or 'abused'. They were 'skewered', 'trussed up like an oven-ready turkey', or treated like a 'slab of meat' or a 'heap of old fish'.[31] When women are handled, perhaps penetrated, in a restraining or punitive way, those who have suffered previous sexual abuse may suffer flashbacks to that abuse.

Hyoscine in the form of scopalamine or 'twilight sleep' was introduced to American hospitals in the second decade of the 20th century. It is a hypnotic drug which makes women unable to remember what happened during childbirth. After it is injected many women become restless, highly excitable and lose all mental control. The woman who has been 'scoped' may fling herself around so much that she is in danger of harming herself. So labouring women were placed in barred, high-sided, padded cots. An obstetrician described her method of restraining patients: 'As the pains increase in frequency and strength, the patient tosses or throws herself about, but without injury to herself, and may be left without fear that she

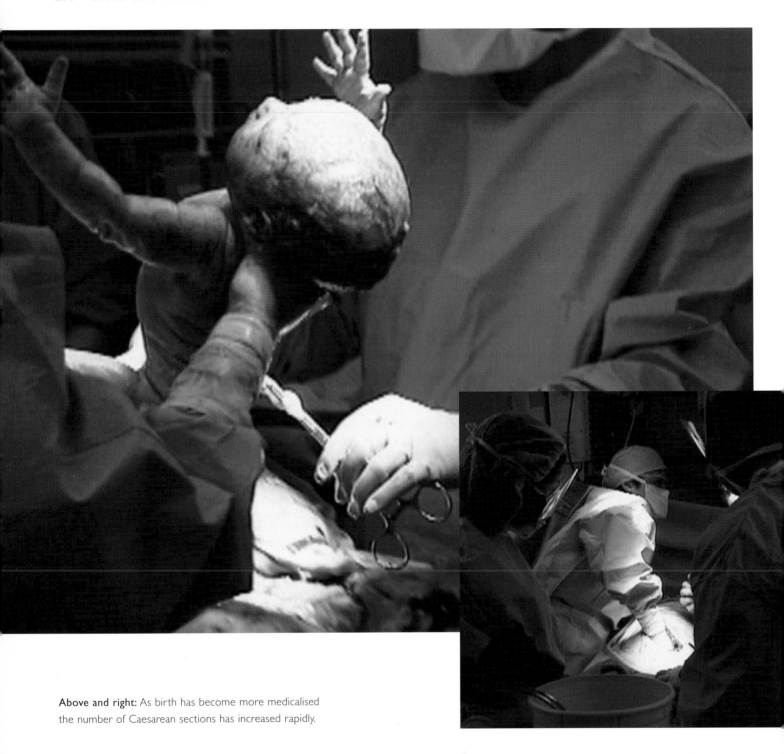

Above and right: As birth has become more medicalised
the number of Caesarean sections has increased rapidly.

will roll on to the floor or be found wandering aimlessly in the corridors. In rare cases, where the patient is very excitable and insists on getting out of bed . . . I prefer to fasten a canvas cover over the tops of the screens, thereby shutting out the light, noise and possibility of leaving the bed.'[32] In some hospitals women wore a kind of baseball helmet to prevent them beating their heads against the sides of the bed and causing brain damage.

An alternative system was the use of a strait jacket. Dr Michelle Harrison, who wrote about her experiences when training in Boston in the 1960s, said:

When these women thought they were 'out' they were awake and screaming. Made crazy from the drug, they fought, they growled like animals, they had to be restrained, tied by hands and feet to the corners of the bed (with straps padded with lambs' wool so there would be no injury, no tell-tale marks) or they would run screaming down the halls. Screaming obscenities, they bit, they wept, behaving in ways that would have produced shame and humiliation had they been aware. Doctors and nurses, looking at such behaviour induced by the drug they had administered, felt justified in treating the women as crazy wild animals to be tied, ordered, slapped, yelled at, gagged.[33]

Scopalamine is still in use in some American hospitals.

It was the custom to leave women fettered on delivery tables for long stretches of time. Protest started in *The Ladies' Home Journal* in 1958.[34] Mothers described horrific experiences: 'When my baby was ready the delivery room wasn't. I was strapped to a table, my legs tied together, so I could "wait" until a more convenient and "safer" time to deliver'; 'I was strapped to a table, hands down, knees up, I remember screaming, "Help me! Help me!" to a nurse who was sitting at a nearby desk. She ignored me'; 'I was strapped to the delivery room table on Saturday morning and lay there until I was delivered on Sunday afternoon.'

As new equipment was developed, manual restraint became increasingly unnecessary and the nurse could concentrate on performing her duties to the obstetrician. Delivery tables were designed with handcuffs, ankle cuffs attached to lithotomy stirrups, and shoulder restrainers on either side of the patient's neck to prevent her raising her head and shoulders from the table. Restraining *touch* gave way to restraining *apparatus*.

In the 1980s, with the electronic revolution in obstetrics, catheters and wires connected to electronic machinery also took the place of human hands, and the use of spinal, caudal and epidural anaesthesia ensured that patients did not toss and turn or move away when an examination or manoeuvre was attempted. The woman was fixed like a laboratory specimen under bright lights, or like an offering on an altar, as gowned and masked professionals conducted the delivery in a shrine-like theatre where the obstetrician served as high priest in the drama of birth.

After the Birth

Greeting touch is practised in most cultures. It consists of contact between hands, arms, lips and cheeks or other parts of the face. This kind of touch is invariably ritualised and differs according to the relative status and relationships of the people greeting each other. The Maori touch noses; in many cultures hand shaking is the norm; in other cultures kissing takes place but only between women; in others men kiss too; the Japanese bow but do not touch.

Everywhere, the newborn baby is greeted with touch – it may be the touch of the obstetrician, the midwife, the mother, the grandmother, the father, and sometimes others. This touch is also ritualised. Within the medical model of birth, the conventional way for an obstetrician to handle the newborn used to be to hold the baby upside down by its ankles and slap it on the bottom. In many traditional cultures throughout the world, birth is followed almost immediately by massage, moulding of the baby's head, 'straightening' of limbs and whole body massage. The baby is bathed or oiled, or both, and then firmly swaddled. Research in the United States has shown that when a mother has the opportunity to hold her unclothed baby immediately after birth, she touches and explores the baby in a spontaneous way that is strikingly different from the ritualised touch of other birth attendants. It has a definite sequence: she first touches the baby lightly with her fingertips and gently pokes the arms and legs. After four or five minutes she strokes the baby's body with the palm of her hand, and at this point becomes excited.[35]

I have often noticed that the new mother usually strokes the fine down or tight curls on the baby's head, traces the lines of the cheeks and nose, and then, as her confidence grows, feels the firmness of the limbs and squeezes the streamlined little bottom. She does something else, too. She brings her face close to the baby and smells it. Her nostrils dilate and she 'breathes in' its reality.

When babies who had been in an intensive care nursery for three weeks (during which time mothers were not allowed to hold them) were at last handed to their mothers, the women touched their babies quite differently. The researchers commented that they 'looked as if they were picking fleas off their babies.'[36]

In my own research on the meeting of mother and baby, if women had received 100 milligrams or more of pethidine (an opiate drug) during labour they often reported that they felt too unsteady to hold their babies safely and did not want to be left alone with them. If the mother did hold her baby she might say, 'I felt drugged'; 'I was too tired to hold her'; 'I was afraid I might drop her'; or 'I wasn't at all interested in seeing the baby. All I wanted to do was go to sleep.'

Almost everywhere in the world birth is followed by massage of the mother and the baby and the application of heat. In India the *dai* massages the sides of the mother's uterus to ensure that all 'dark blood' and clots (*gandagi*) flow back to the earth from whence they came. The rich blood that nurtured

Right: Everywhere, the newborn baby is greeted by touch. But the way in which the child is touched by care-givers varies enormously.

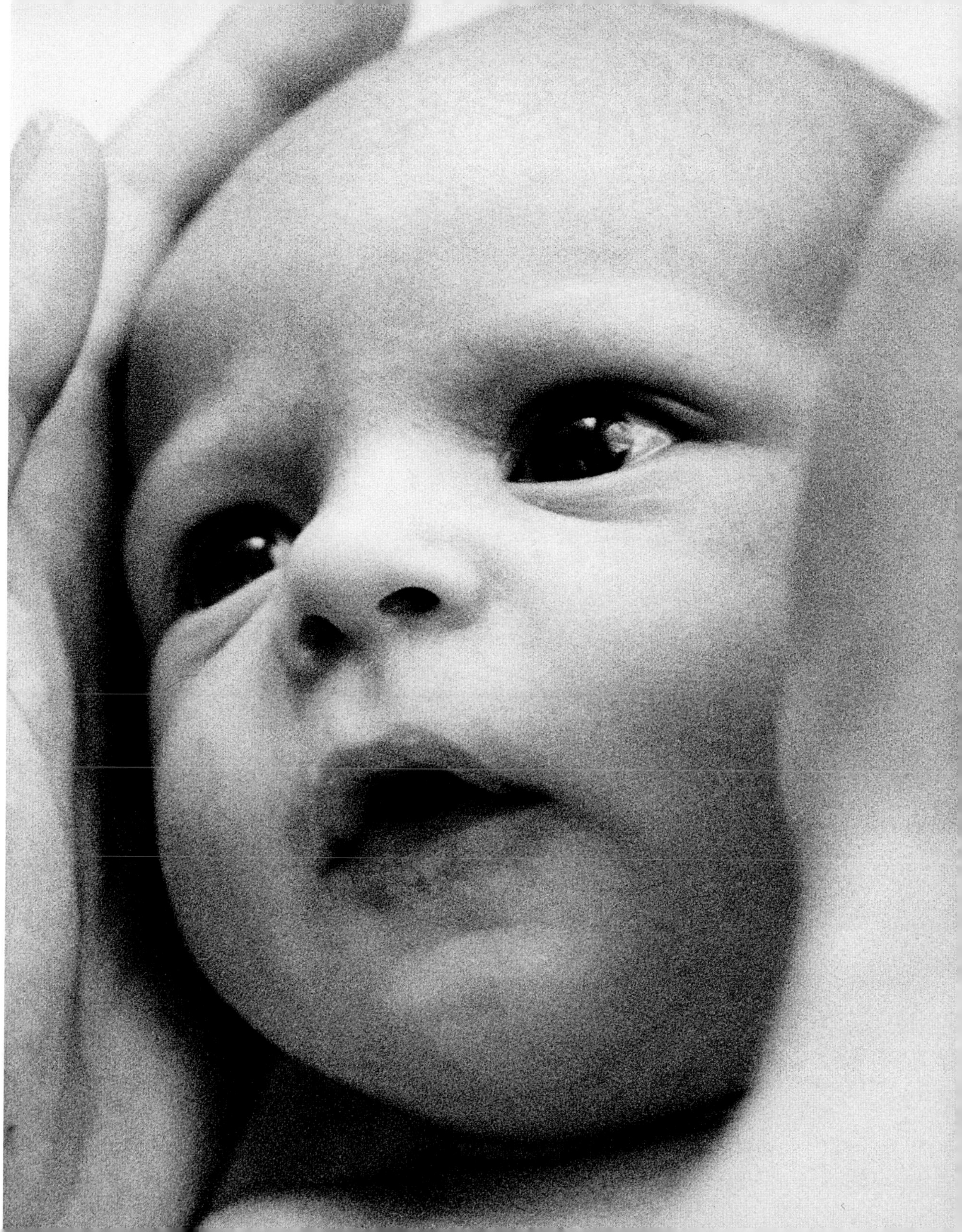

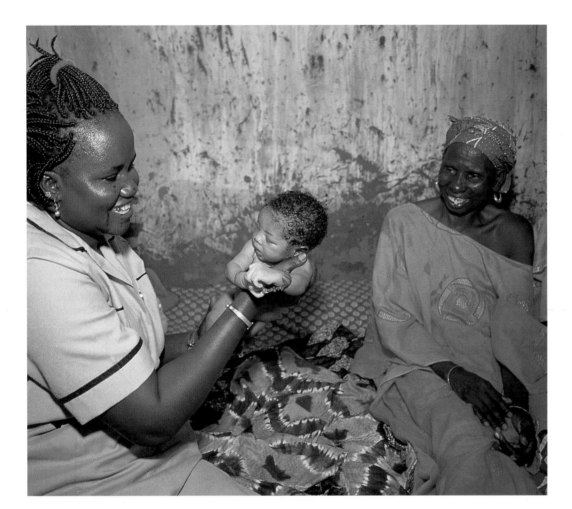

the baby within the uterus is personified as the Goddess Bemata, meaning 'mother's love'. Once the child is born she comes down seeking the baby she has lost and this is a dangerous phase of birth. Good blood has become 'bad blood'. The uterus must be encouraged to contract and to involute, and bleeding is welcomed as a sign that this is happening. To retain clots and polluting dark blood inside the uterus is to risk death. Massage enables blood to flow freely and the woman's open body to become closed.

The placenta is considered the sibling or the 'mother' of the child. It is invariably handled with respect, and often reverence, for it is the baby's tree of life, and it is ritually buried or burned. When a woman dies after childbirth it is because this has not happened and the placenta, which is the 'other mother', has 'gone up' and killed her.

In most cultures the umbilical cord is not cut until the baby is breathing.

The traveller Verrier Elwin quotes from a description of a birth in the Maikal hills: 'Life passed through the cord into the flower (the placenta) and the child went cold. We brought two handfuls of grass from the roof and placed the flower on it and lit it. As the flower grew warm, life flowed back into the child.'[37] Heating the placenta caused placental blood to flow into the baby. To achieve this in Burma the placenta is sometimes placed in a frying pan over the fire.

In Guatemala, the midwife gives a general massage to stimulate the mother's circulation, massages her legs, and then 'closes' the pelvis with a binder. Polynesian and Melanesian women massage the mother's abdomen and start a fire of dried coconut fronds to give her warmth, since immediately after birth she is in a 'cold' state. This is so not only in terms of metaphysical theories of hot and cold; a newly delivered mother is often shivering and welcomes warmth. In Malaysia, the Philippines and the Solomon Islands, the midwife swaddles the mother's abdomen and lower back with heated leaves.[38] A Zuni woman wears a strip of cloth holding in place a heated stone. The Kwakiutl of British Columbia use heated kelp, pressing it against the new mother's abdomen and in the small of her back.[39] In both Australia and North America the mother rests on a heated sand bed, while in California, Native American women lie in beds in a pit lined with stones that have been heated in a fire, with sand over the stones. Sometimes the mother is buried up to the armpits and knees in warm sand instead.

Massage is continued through the postpartum days, and sometimes for much longer. Malaysian midwives use a 'hot' mixture of salt, turmeric or ginger, lime and tamarind ground into a paste. This is not restricted to women who have traditional births; even those who are delivered in hospital look forward to this massage once they are home again. The midwife visits for the first three days after birth to give a complete body massage. In northern India, too, the *dai* massages the woman's abdomen, arms and legs each day. Midwives in Thailand massage for a full month after childbirth using the yellow sap from the cumin tree, and explain that this massage is needed to 'help the womb enter its cradle', because it encourages the uterus to contract, become smaller and firmer, and sink back into the pelvic cavity.[40]

A new mother in Santa Lucia, Guatemala, takes sweat baths every three or four days and may receive a massage while she is in the bath. Or she squats over a pail of steaming hot water to which some milk and special herbs have been added. This is similar to Jamaican practice, where *nanas* recommend steaming the perineum over a bucket of water which must be 'hot like nine nights' love'.[41] Sometimes herbal baths are taken instead. The midwife gives the new mother an abdominal massage, and may also massage her legs if she thinks there is risk of varicose veins. She then repositions the binder around her pelvic area so as to put pressure over the uterus and 'close the bones'.[42]

The ritualised *fire rest* is a normal element in postnatal care throughout Burma, Thailand and Vietnam. In south-east Asia, when a house is built a wood is planted 'so that every generation of occupants would have it available for use at confinements'.[43] In Vietnam, the mother lies with a small charcoal burning stove or heated bricks under the planks of her bed for one month after the birth and takes a steam bath every day.

It was customary for the Thai mother to stay in a special birth room for one or two weeks after birth. Four planks of banana tree wood were laid in squares around the wall of her room and formed a frame for a fire. She lay on this on her side, wearing only a loin cloth. In the 19th century, Queen Prabporapak, whose doctors were English, criticised this practice, established a medical school and paid women to go into hospital to give birth, where they were offered hot water bottles instead of the fire rests. Mothers had to wait until they got home to continue the traditional ritual. The fire rest is not only an Eastern custom. Traditionally, the newly delivered Jewish mother rested beside a fire for up to thirty days after the birth, including on the Sabbath, when work such as the lighting of fires was otherwise forbidden.

In many countries hot compresses are also applied over the uterus. In India these may be bags of sand or dried and powdered cow dung. In Thailand they consist of heated salt in a cloth bag.[44] Among the Ainu, an

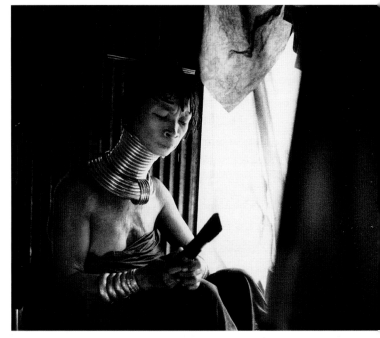

Above: A Kayan woman in Thailand has saunas for three days after birth.

aboriginal people in Japan, the hot salt is placed in a small basket and pressed against the uterus, or hot bricks are used. Throughout the Caribbean stones may be heated and employed for this purpose, as in Malaysia where a smooth, flat stone is placed against the new mother's abdomen.

Heat in the form of herbal vapour or smoke is also used to help the mother's perineum heal after childbirth. In the Yemen the perineum may be fomented with essential oils every day. The midwife prepares a brazier and sprinkles on frankincense and myrrh and holds it beneath the woman's skirts so that the smoke envelops her perineum. There, as in the Caribbean, fomentation is thought to be the best method of cleaning the vulva and, with the addition of herbs or other natural substances, enabling it to heal. It is probably a much more hygienic method than handling the tissues with soap and water.

The idea threading through these virtually worldwide customs of heat and massage is that the uterus needs to be held, supported and warmed. This is achieved either by the local application of heat, by firm binding, or both as in Malaysia, Japan, North Africa, South America, the Caribbean and, until the 1930s, in many parts of Europe. My mother, who was a midwife in the years after the First World War, described to me how she bound the new mother's body firmly with wide strips of cloth from below the breasts to the top of the legs. Each time the midwife visited in the days following the birth she unwound the cloth strips, gave the mother a bed-bath, patted her dry, and then rebound her. She offered the intimate and nurturing touch which was considered an important part of postnatal care. In modern hospitals new mothers are rarely touched except to examine them to check that the uterus is firm and, if they had an episiotomy or tear, to examine the perineum.

In traditional cultures there is strong focus on the physical elements of mothering in the first postpartum weeks, on prolonged skin contact between mother and baby, oiling and massage, and firm binding with strips of cloth. These are primarily tactile experiences; to them are added the psycho-physiological effects of heat, fire and steam bathing.

In modern hospitals the smells are usually of antiseptic, cleaning detergent, institutional floor polish, perhaps a whiff of baby powder and the mothers' deodorants, hairsprays, perfumes and make-up. Smells of blood, amniotic fluid, sweat and breastmilk are eradicated. Mothers and babies may never be able to smell each other under these conditions. Yet we know that a baby at birth has a keen sense of smell and can find its way to the breast by scent alone. We know, too, that each baby prefers the scent of its own mother's breast to any other mother's.

The traditional lying-in room is small and dark, infused by the scents of birth and postbirth. The mother and the women tending her are physically close. She is caressed, cradled, stroked. The fire's embers glow, hot fomentations spiked with herbs and essential oils make her flesh soft and damp. There are smells of hot soup, chicken and porridge, the ritual nourishment of parturition. It is a sensory experience far removed from the sights, smells and sounds of a modern hospital.

From the vantage point of our own technological culture, the traditional postpartum experience is much more physical. It is also intensely sensual. The mother has her baby close to her and holds, touches, strokes, massages and explores the baby, breathing in this child who has been born from her body. She in turn is held, touched, stroked, massaged and cherished by those who share her journey into motherhood.

There may be something that we can learn from traditional patterns of nurturing the new mother and baby, and from the tactile experiences which could facilitate and enrich the postpartum experience for women today.

Chapter 8

Sanctuary and Renewal

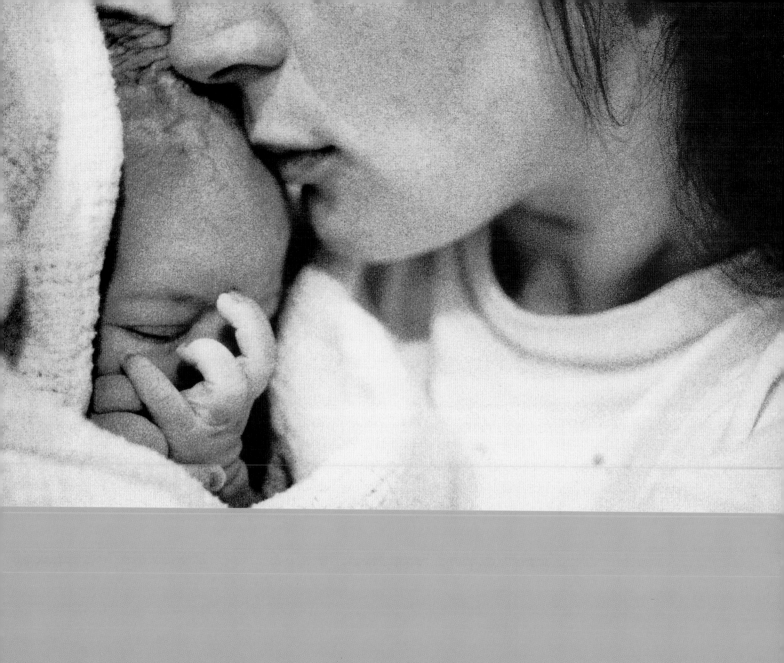

In many cultures the newborn baby is thought of as hovering between the spirit world of the ancestors and the world of here and now. A baby is in a state of becoming. Its soul has not settled firmly into the little body.

When a newborn baby in Zimbabwe is not thriving the traditional midwife may diagnose a breast-feeding problem and give the mother herbs to stimulate her milk supply, but she will also 'talk to the spirits'. This is why women who give birth in hospital still choose to receive after-care from a midwife who is possessed by one or more spirits of her dead family members. Hospitals and clinics offer physical care, but spiritual protection can only be provided by a midwife who consults spirits with whom she has a special relationship. The decision to become a midwife was in itself a result of being called to her vocation by these spirits.[1]

An important part of the preparation for birth is often the creation of ritual objects that will be hung in different places around the house following the birth to ward off evil spirits. In Sarawak the father makes bamboo crosses to be placed above the lying-in bed (the *nangkat*) on which the mother has her *fire rest*, at the side of the ladder of the stilted longhouse which is shared by several families, and anywhere else where malevolent spirits could attack the mother or baby.[2]

If a Jamaican baby is allowed to cry, a *duppy*, who is often the spirit of a grandmother or other female relative who has died, will come to comfort it and feel unable to part with it. As a result, the baby will sicken and may die. A newborn is protected from this possessive spirit love during the transitional forty days after birth by having the Bible left open at the 23rd Psalm, a pair of scissors and a tape measure beside it if the mother has to turn her back or leave the baby unattended, even for a few minutes. She dresses the baby in something red, because *duppies* dislike this colour, and bathes it in water containing washing blue which keeps *duppies* away. She may also burn incense in order to attract the angels. Should a baby be at special risk, she obtains a bag of charms from an *obeah* (a sorcerer) and fixes it to the baby's clothing.

A Hopi baby's face is not uncovered until twenty days after birth, lest its spirit escape through its mouth. At that time the mother lifts the blanket and introduces the baby to the sun and to the life-giving spirit of corn, the staple food of the Hopi, with a brief prayer. Only after this does she take the baby to visit families in the community.

Babies are almost invariably kept indoors for at least a week after birth, and often, as in Jamaica, in a darkened room with doors and windows closed to give them special protection. Only when the umbilical cord stump falls off is a Ngoni baby in Malawi ready to leave the hut for the first time. Then the child is presented to the village in a ceremony that takes place in the late afternoon, as the men are coming home from work, so that they can 'salute the new stranger'.[3]

The new mother is also passing through a stage of transition. They are each on a bridge into the unknown; it is a time of spiritual and physiological risk and metamorphosis. Both mother and baby are seen as in an 'in-between' state of being, in which they require special protection and nurturing. This is particularly marked when a woman gives birth to her first child, but it happens to some extent with the birth of every baby.

Following the birth, the womb must have time to 'enter its cradle' again (the Thai term for the involution of the uterus and its descent into the pelvis), and the woman's spine must 'knit up' (a Jamaican phrase). In Thailand, as in Jamaica, the midwife visits to massage the mother every day to assist this process, relieve muscle pain and help her get her figure back. The Indian *dai* visits the mother's house twice a day to do this, using a mixture of oil and turmeric to massage both mother and baby. Most cultures have their own version of baby massage to help the limbs grow straight and strong, to shape the head so that it is beautiful, and to relieve any digestive or other discomfort the baby may be experiencing. The massage of the mother is often followed by the binding of her abdomen with cloth; the baby is often swaddled after massage, too.

The changes taking place for both mother and baby are not only physical. They are spiritual and social. In most cultures the weeks immediately following birth are a time of protection, hedged around with specific dietary and other rules which require the active co-operation of the various women in the family and neighbourhood. It is a time when women friends gather together to care for and cherish mother and baby and, as we saw in Chapter 4, to reaffirm female bonds of loyalty and love. Only in extremes of poverty or social isolation are women expected to get back to work – cooking, cleaning, labouring on the land and carrying heavy loads – shortly after childbirth. Usually there is a period of sanctuary, a virtual holiday, when the clamour of demands made on a woman is stilled, when she can just be. In traditional cultures it is rare for most women to have this space in their lives, and it is all the more precious when it comes with the birth of a baby.

The 'lying-in' that our own grandmothers experienced represents the surviving vestige of a system of seclusion following birth in which a new mother in this marginal social and spiritual state remained islanded with her baby for a set period of time. A statutory ten-day 'lying-in' period was implemented following the 1902 Midwives' Act in Britain, and was the basis for the midwife visiting the home for ten days after the birth.

The pattern of seclusion of mother and baby, and their nurturing by women close to them, is found all over the world. It is commonly forty days, a period in which a woman is exempt from her usual tasks and receives nourishing food and support. Traditionally, it has been an important factor both for the survival of the newborn and for the 'tuning in' and emotional bonding of mother and baby, and remains the ritual ideal in many cultures.

In many traditional societies the woman who has just emerged from childbirth, whose body is 'open' and from whom blood is issuing, is considered in a marginal state of existence, which makes her vulnerable and tender. But she is also unclean, and particularly threatening to men. As a result she is sometimes almost totally isolated, and in rural areas of India, for example, food is passed through an opening under the door.

In southern India the Adivi mother used to be in a state of complete ritual seclusion. She stayed with her baby in a hut made of leaves and mats for ninety days, while her husband built a hut nearby and watched over her. If anyone touched her they were expelled from the village for three months.

In traditional Chinese medicine, harmony must be maintained between 'hot' and 'cold'. Women are 'Yin' and have more of a 'cold' in their nature than men. So they are particularly susceptible to illness resulting from cold. In pregnancy a woman is especially cold, whereas the fetus is hot and this causes 'wind' to be generated in her body. During the monthly cycle the woman oscillates between 'hot' in the mid-cycle to 'cold' when she is menstruating. Both menstrual blood and blood following childbirth are dirty and must flow freely or they cause illness.

A Chinese woman is not supposed to leave her home while she 'does the month', that is from the birth until the moon has passed through a full cycle. The character for 'month' and that for 'moon' is the same. She stays in her 'month room', does not wash dishes or do laundry, and must avoid cold water at all costs as it causes wind to enter her body, leading to rheumatism and other illnesses later in life. When she washes, the water is first brought to the boil then cooled. Mugwort or fresh ginseng and pomelo leaves may be boiled with it first. She does not take a bath or swim during this period.

Chinese women have heard that women in the West get straight out of bed after childbirth 'like hens laying eggs'.

If she decides to leave the house she must do so with great caution, wearing a hat or carrying an umbrella to protect her head, or taking care to stay in the shade, for she must avoid sun as well as wind. There must be no air conditioning or draughts in the home for it is thought that all the joints in her body are open after childbirth. Similarly, air conditioning is turned off in maternity hospitals even on hot days.

The new mother stays in bed as much as possible, lying flat on her back, so that her spine can mend. Chinese women have heard that women in the West get straight out of bed after childbirth 'like hens laying eggs'.[4] She must also be careful not to strain her eyes. If she reads she may have problems with her eyesight in the future. Sexual intercourse during this time is considered very dangerous, for the man as well as the woman, and may lead to all kinds of illness.

When she reaches the end of this seclusion period there is a celebration and the family gathers to drink the 'full month wine'.

Ritual practices enacted through fear can turn into an ordeal. An eighty-one-year-old Chinese woman, who gave birth in her maternal village, describes what happened to her:

I could not lie down. Otherwise blood would go to the upper part of my body. I had to sit on the bed for nearly 24 hours. I also could not close my eye-lids to sleep. Otherwise I would get cold. If I would close my eye-lids my mother awake me. I must sit and not sleep nearly 24 hours. I must keep warm and use cloth band wrapped my forehead [sic] to beware of headache afterwards.

When the husband's mother provides most of the help around the birth, one result of the ritual of 'doing the month' is that a woman and her mother-in-law are usually drawn closer together. Until a woman has her first baby she is almost on sufferance in her husband's family. The baby's birth, especially if the child is male, confirms her status as a family member and there is a relaxation of tension and pressure. An anthropologist describes it in this way:

Under such circumstances, 'doing the month' is clearly a reward, and an important role reversal takes place. Having been obliged from the day of marriage to wait hand and foot on and be at the beck and call of her mother-in-law, the mother of the newborn infant is now given sanction to lie idle in bed for an entire month – waited upon and pampered by the mother-in-law herself.[5]

Similar seclusion, though usually not extended for such a length of time, is common in cultures all over the world. In North America, the tradition was that a Hopi mother and baby remained in a darkened room for eighteen days. Each day a mark was made on the wall and an ear of corn placed beneath it. On the nineteenth day the mother ground all this corn for the ceremony of purification and celebration that took place on the following day. For most north-west coast natives there was a twelve-day seclusion, shared with both the husband and the helping women.

A Mexican woman in Yucatan is secluded for seven days in a room sealed from outside influences so that bad spirits cannot enter. Doors and windows are shut, and any cracks stuffed with rags. She emerges twenty days after birth, when the *partera* makes her last postpartum visit, gives her a massage, the *sobada*, and then firmly binds her abdomen and pelvis with a girdle, the *faja*. She will wear this girdle for as long as she feels the need; because peasant women have to carry heavy loads, she may wear it all the time. The period of seclusion is ended at twenty days, since the Mayan calendar was divided into twenty-day segments. It has been suggested that the 260-day year, divided into thirteen twenty-day months, is based on the length of human pregnancy.[6]

In Uganda, the Acholi woman keeps to her house for three days if she has delivered a boy, four days if it is a girl, and is cared for by either her mother or her husband's mother. It is thought that if anyone else crosses the threshold the baby will get ill or become blind, or the mother become infertile.

A new mother in Jamaica is considered at risk of *baby chill*, in much the same way as the Chinese woman. She should not wash her hair for forty days after the birth and must keep it done up in a turban. Though in practice she may not be able to do this, the ideal is that she rests to enable the gateway in her lower spine, which opened to let the baby out, to 'knit up' again. It is usually a woman in her own family who looks after her, either her mother or an aunt or older sister. Failing that, the help of a neighbour.

In Europe, gypsy culture treats a new mother as polluted for several weeks, and she has her own special tent and crockery. At the end of the period of seclusion her tent and bedding are ritually burned, but she is still not allowed to prepare food for men for some weeks following.

The new Jewish mother was traditionally cared for entirely by other women for thirty days after birth. They built a fire close by her and tended it even on the Sabbath, when work like this was usually forbidden, and she was plied with nourishing dishes.

In the Middle Ages there was a good deal of theological argument within the Christian church about whether it was right to seclude women and prohibit them from attending religious services following childbirth. Pope Gregory told St Augustine: 'This is to be understood as an allegory, for were a woman to enter church and return thanks in the very hour of her delivery she would do no wrong.' The effect of the allegory was that the new mother was freed from her usual services as a wife, and instead was tended by her god-sibs. It is clear that seclusion is interpreted differently in different cultures. In the majority of cultures, however, seclusion simply implies that there is no contact with men. It is a time for women to come together. The mother rests and other women visit her, bringing gifts and admiring the baby. It is a great social occasion.

Lying-in Foods

In all societies new mothers are provided with special food. These are foods intended to make the woman strong and to increase her milk supply, while others are taboo. The woman whose body is open and from whom blood and lochia is issuing is 'cold', so she eats 'hot' foods – not literally hot, but those that generate inner vitality and which balance the coldness in her body. In Malaysia, for example, she is given dried fish, rice, cassava, spices, bread, bananas, durian, rambutan and milk. Eggs should be eaten every day, mixed with honey, pepper and yeast, and beef for those who can afford it. In Jamaica the nanas emphasise the importance of good nutrition after birth and advise the new mother to eat rice, soup, potato, chocho, fresh meat and chicken and to drink cerasee tea (often called 'bitters') because 'it clean and bring the blood'. The aim is to ensure that no 'bad' blood remains trapped in the body, a belief remarkably similar to that of Indian *dais*.

The new mother does not eat 'cold' or raw foods. Cold foods include turnips, Chinese cabbage, bamboo shoots, green leafy vegetables, most fruit, and duck and fish, because they live in water. Drinking iced water is considered particularly dangerous. A Chinese woman now in her eighties says that in the first seven days after birth she had to be particularly careful of her diet, avoid highly salted and oily foods, and eat small quantities of pulses, chicken soup and bean curd.

Some foods are particularly suitable in the first month. In Taiwan, sesame seed chicken is the special dish eaten while 'sitting out the month.' It is cooked in sesame oil and rice wine. In the People's Republic of China the chicken is prepared with dates. Chicken soup, chicken liver and kidneys, pork liver and eggs are good, too, resulting in a very high protein diet for the mother.

Other foods that have the effect of flushing out 'dirty blood' are fermented rice with eggs, rice wine infused with ginger, offal and noodles in brown sugar. Salt is bad, but sweet food is good, including sweet chicken and porridge with brown sugar. Some foods are believed to be of special help with breastfeeding, specifically pigs' trotters, bream and certain herbs that fall into the category of 'hot'.

Historically in Japan, the mother's food was cooked by female family members exclusively for her in a separate pot over a special fire for thirty-five days following the birth. There was a ceremony of purification to mark the end of this transitional period, and then she immersed herself in the sea or a bath, or she and the baby were sprinkled with salt. Still today Japanese mothers must not visit the shrine for thirty-five days, and babies are rarely taken out of the home until they are about one month old.

Among the Galla of Ethiopia the birth of a baby is celebrated by song, and when the expectant mother returns to her mother's home to give birth she takes with her two, four or six women to help after the birth, one or more of whom must be a good singer. Birth takes place in the back room, *borro*, of the house, with the mother kneeling on freshly strewn grass and supported by her women friends. As soon as the baby is born the women ululate, four times for a girl, five for a boy. They follow this with improvised birth songs proclaiming the mother's gallantry in giving birth, and her happiness, and give thanks to the Maram, the Goddess of Childbirth. They compare the mother's achievement with that of the brave hunter who returns victorious to the village. On the first day the choir sing just two or three of these, but over the next few days they build up to a full repertoire. The atmosphere is light-hearted and relaxed and the singing is punctuated by conversation. An anthropologist who has recorded many of these songs gives a typical example:

Soloist: *O woman with child, it was good you gave birth. (This is taken up by the chorus) . . . Honour adorns your* borro. *Your husband stands at the door laughing. Maram adorned your* borro. *O Maram let me be strong for you. Let me be pleasing to you. Let me gain strength from you. O Maram I have value in your eyes. The hunter returns to the wilderness and the lying-in woman to labour. The hunter should have his spoils. With a buffalo tail he is worth seeing. The woman should have her spoils. With a child she is worth seeing.*
Chorus: *Woman with child it was good you gave birth.*[7]

On the Japanese island of Okinawa, birth is also greeted with song. All the women who have attended the birth welcome the baby and sing, 'May this baby always laugh and be pleasant.'[8]

In diverse cultures the period of puerperal seclusion defines the boundaries of an exclusive and concentrated female social space in which the mother is nurtured by women who draw together in female solidarity. Everything that is done is comfortingly familiar, takes place in a domestic context, and is controlled by women. The time of cherishing, nurturing foods, loving touch and celebration plays an important part in enhancing a woman's self-image after childbirth, and in easing the emotional transition to motherhood. With the male take-over of childbirth, and the professionalisation of care, this has been lost in technocratic culture.

The 'islanding' of mother and baby also has the effect of enhancing the woman's relationship with her baby. In preindustrial societies the general pattern of care is that a baby stays close by the mother day and night, often fixed to her body, bound by shawls, slung in a net or other carrier, or wound in a strip of cloth. Because a baby is carried close to the body the mother can respond instantly. This close physical contact continues for some months after birth. The physical connection with the mother is considered so essential that in some African cultures the cloth that attaches the baby to its mother's back is called the 'placenta'. Life outside the uterus is treated as a continuation of life inside it. In many cultures the baby is shielded from danger under the mother's clothing, in flesh to flesh contact.

There is no breastfeeding schedule, no timing of feeds or the interval between them. The baby is fed

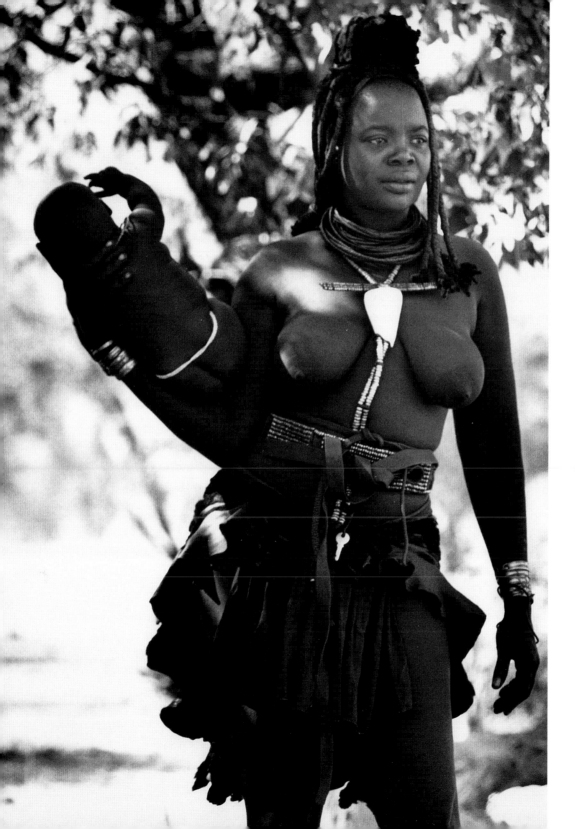

Left: A Himba mother and her baby in Namibia.

freely throughout the twenty-four hours. Access to the breast is unrestricted. In Yucatan, for example, a baby is never set down to go to sleep and is placed in the hammock only after it is already asleep. As soon as the baby starts to wake the breast is offered. The mother's breast, or in some societies another woman's, is offered whenever it stirs. A study in Papua New Guinea revealed that throughout the night women never had an interval in suckling of longer than twenty minutes.

When interviewing in traditional societies I have often found it difficult to explain to mothers that this is not so everywhere in the world, for they say that of course babies must be close to their mother's bodies; of course they must be fed whenever they seek the breast, for how else can they survive, and who else can the baby possibly belong to? I met with reactions of disbelief from women shocked to hear that in the West, immediately after birth, a baby is often separated from the mother and put in a nursery where it is looked after by people who are not even related to her.

Other striking exceptions exist, all the more noticeable because they are discordant with a traditional pattern of mother and baby togetherness. Among some urban families in Taiwan the mother returns home to 'do the month' while the baby stays in hospital, being returned to the family at the end of the month. In some families too, the mother-in-law takes over the baby and the mother is left to rest and recuperate by herself.[9] Bonding takes place between the baby and the grandmother. Bonding between mother and baby is treated as of less importance. This may be one reason why breastfeeding is declining in China. With the one child policy, older women can look forward to having only one or two grandchildren. The grandmother role has always been central to family and community life there. So the proud grandmother takes over care of the baby, whom she bottle-feeds while the mother first 'keeps the month', but without her baby beside her, and then returns to work.

In Yucatan a baby is never set down to go to sleep and is placed in the hammock only after it is already asleep. As soon as the baby starts to wake the breast is offered.

'Welcome To Our Family'

It is acknowledged good practice in infant care to put the baby to the mother's breast within an hour of birth and to breastfeed exclusively. Newborn babies do not need other foods and fluids. Research in industrialised countries reveals that giving anything other than breastmilk reduces the chances of successful breastfeeding[10]. It can also be dangerous, because alien foods and fluids such as sugar destroy the normal bacteria in the baby's intestines and interfere with the immune system.

Yet in many traditional cultures, where virtually all women breastfeed successfully and babies are fed on demand once breastfeeding is established, they may not be put to the breast until the mature milk 'comes in' at three or four days. They are not given colostrum, the first form of milk in the breast, and they may be breastfed by other women during that time, fed prelacteal foods or fluids, or be given something to make them vomit mucus before being put to the breast.

The World Health Organisation (WHO) and UNICEF are concerned to change these practices, and there is a concerted effort by health workers in countries such as India and Pakistan to teach 'traditional birth attendants' (TBAs) that mothers should breastfeed exclusively.

One problem is that when attempts are made to stamp out indigenous cultural practices like these, their social function is ignored or trivialised. Everything that is done in traditional patterns of birth and the care of new babies hangs together. The actions an observer records are not quaint interpretations of ancient superstitions, though they are sometimes written about by health workers trained in the Western medical model who are keen to eradicate harmful practices as if they were just that. Each practice is part of a system of belief and an unwritten script that is embedded in the culture.

As a culture disintegrates or changes rapidly, these customs lose or change their meaning. Often people cling to them because they offer some semblance of order and assurance of continuity, though when confronted with scientific evidence that they are harmful they cannot defend them logically. The result is head-on conflict between two opposed belief systems.

Sometimes these practices are interwoven with religious rites and reinforced by beliefs about divine commandments, the wishes of the ancestors, and the spiritual and cultural heritage of one's people. Indian texts from the 4th century BC to the 1st century AD advised that the newborn baby be given a sanctified mixture of honey, clarified butter, the juices of leaves and roots, and gold dust.[11]

In China, though the mother is 'cold' after giving birth, the baby is considered 'hot' and the first fluid given is intended to remove this heat. A Chinese woman described how her baby was given 'three wong soup', a herbal mixture that includes rhubarb and 'clears unclean things from inside of the baby's body'.

The first breastfeed is often preceded by a mild herbal tea, such as camomile tea in peasant Mexico, though in many cultures it is thought important to make the baby pass meconium as soon as possible, so purgatives are given.

The most popular method is to give butter or almond oil mixed with sugar, honey or syrup. In Jamaica, the *nana* places a few drops of castor oil on the baby's tongue to make it vomit any mucus before being given the breast for the first time. If the mother is working in the fields or 'higgling' at market and the baby cries, another woman will provide mint tea or coconut water. The baby is given another dose of oil nine days after birth. This marks the ritual transition into a full state of existence and away from the dangers of birth.

In many cultures the gift of food or herbal tea to the new baby is a rite that is part of the bonding process between the mother and the womenfolk in her husband's family.

When food or fluid is offered as part of a ceremony enacted by the baby's father it represents acceptance of the baby as his and the taking on of paternal responsibility. The Hindu or the Sikh father does not see his baby's face until the rite takes place in which he puts honey or ghee on the baby's tongue, and the Sikh father whispers words from the holy books. When alternatives to breastmilk are offered by the midwife, this represents a confirmation of her role as a major influence in the child's life and her connectedness with the family.

We need to understand these customs in terms of the reinforcement of relationships, for the social effect of such practices is to engage other women in the group in the active care of mother and baby. They have a cohesive function. The baby is not simply the child of its biological mother, but the child of a group of women linked in commitment to each other.

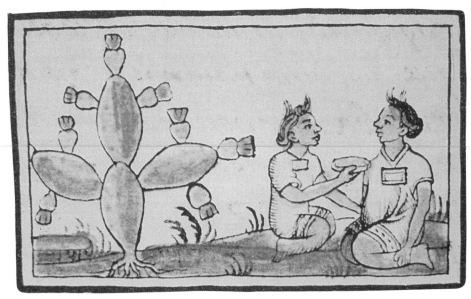

Right: In Mexico, in the Mayan tradition, a herbal tea is given to the mother to help her breastfeed.

Bonding

Some research papers treat bonding as if it were a magic glue that sticks mother and baby together, regardless of the environment and regardless of the kind of care that is given to a mother. It is considered an automatic mechanism triggered by the sight of the baby. Bonding is studied in isolation, as if there were no relationship between the way birth is conducted – all that has preceded those moments of meeting – and the mother's first sight of her newborn. Doctor Aidan Macfarlane has recorded the meeting of mothers and babies on video tape, and reveals that there is a wide variation in the degree to which mothers feel free to touch and explore their babies, and that this is associated with the

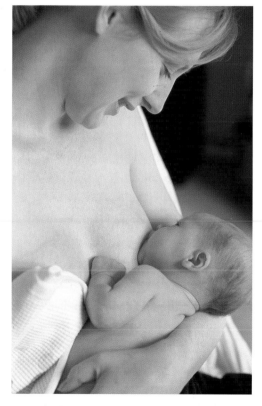

relationship between a woman and her midwife. When certain midwives assisted at the birth there was more expression of emotion and more flesh to flesh contact between mother and baby, not because the midwife told the mother that this should be done, but because she provided an environment in which the woman was able to express spontaneously whatever she felt. The quality of emotional support given by a midwife, and her warmth of character, may be an important element in enabling a woman to reach out to her baby and fall in love with it.

There is an enormous difference between the first days of life in a peasant culture and the beginning of life in many modern maternity hospitals. The mother has had to move out of her home, the equivalent of the mother animal's nest, into the hospital, and must often give birth among strangers. Her body is treated as a container to be emptied of its contents. She is processed through childbirth as if the fetus were a manufactured product, put together, monitored and packaged on a factory assembly line. She may feel that her body no longer belongs to her, but functions only because of things done to it by professional care-givers. For some women the result is a massive loss of self-confidence, a sense of failure, and dependency on their care-givers.[12] This is one reason for the emotional crisis that often follows home-coming, when for the first time a woman must take responsibility for her baby and interpret its cues appropriately. Not only has she been alienated from her own body, she has also been alienated from her baby.

In many countries this sense of alienation is further aggravated by separation of the mother and her baby. In the United States, as in Russia and Eastern European countries, babies continue to be removed to a nursery immediately following delivery for up to twelve hours, and while the mother remains on the postpartum ward she may be allowed to have her baby with her only at scheduled feed times. I have witnessed births in Russia, the Czech Republic and Poland after which women are not even permitted to hold and touch their babies lest bacteria be conveyed to the baby, and hence to the communal nursery. Babies remain in the nursery for the whole of the hospital stay, which may be as long as ten days after a Caesarean section.

WHO and UNICEF have introduced the Baby Friendly Hospital Initiative, but even in hospitals designated as 'baby friendly' some separation may still be the norm. The mother puts the baby to the breast six to eight hours after birth, depending on the hospital time-table, and the baby is 'topped up' with formula milk. Women have to 'empty' their breasts after each feed with the help of a breast pump, even while babies are being given supplementary bottle feeds. Engorgement and mastitis are common as a result of this practice. Feeds are given by schedule, and babies are wheeled to their mothers on multi-baby trolleys at the designated times. If they cry between feeds they are given water or glucose water. Mothers are not allowed to care for their babies. Changing and bathing must be done by midwives, nurses or maternal child nurses. Mothers are often required to wear hats, masks and protective garments while breastfeeding, and sometimes to put a plastic sheet between themselves and their babies.[13]

They must often wash their breasts or spray them with antiseptic, and the baby's mouth may be washed out with antiseptic before each feed and the lips painted with gentian violet or another form of antiseptic. The mother's finger may also be sprayed or painted with antiseptic. Feeding times are limited and mothers are taught to extend these times gradually and often to use nipple shields. Free samples of nipple shields and formula milk are often provided in postpartum 'baby boxes'.

In countries where rooming-in is allowed after vaginal birth, babies are often still routinely removed to the nursery following Caesarean. One in six mothers in the UK and one in four in the USA now has a Caesarean section. Private patients everywhere have more Caesarean sections than those in any national health scheme. In Brazil, for example, 90 per cent of private patients are delivered by Caesarean section, compared with 25 per cent of clinic patients. So the most privileged mothers are the most deprived when it comes to contact with their babies.

In a technocratic culture, the six weeks after childbirth are treated as a time for medical processing and for speedy social adjustment. The new mother should demonstrate that 'she has got her figure back' within a few weeks. The aim is for a woman to return to normal as quickly as possible, and to fit the baby into her life. Great value is set on independence, and a baby often only a few days old is expected to be

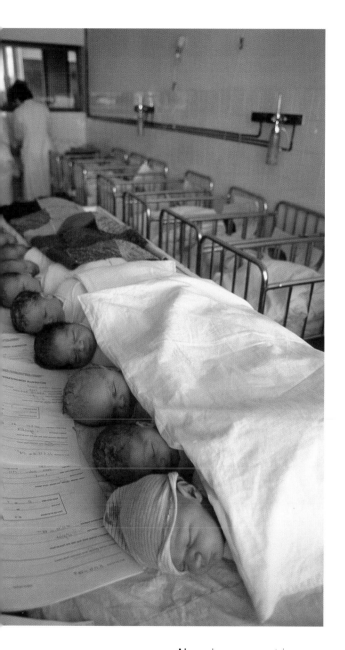

Above: In some countries babies are still removed to a nursery immediately following birth.

as independent as possible, to sleep in its own cot, to manage three or four hours regularly between feeds, not to wake at night, and to comfort and amuse itself.

I once heard a consultant obstetrician who objected to Frederick Leboyer's teaching about 'gentle birth' declare in a lecture, 'Life is cold and hard. The sooner a child starts to learn that, the better. Why not at birth?' He expressed succinctly the very opposite belief as to how newborn babies should be cared for to that found in traditional cultures all over the world.

Babies are rarely left to cry. In fact, they may not cry at all. In Africa, !Kung babies are picked up and given the breast without delay whenever they stir. Research reveals that in 92 per cent of fussing or crying episodes they are attended to within fifteen seconds; the average time is six seconds.[14] These babies are fed, on average, four times an hour for three years or longer. They are in physical contact with their mothers or another care-giver 90 per cent of the time during the day, and in the night sleep beside their parents. It has been calculated that, in contrast, babies in northern industrialised countries are allowed to cry from five to thirty minutes before anyone does anything about it. It is sometimes claimed that crying is 'good' for them because it makes them expand their lungs. Or it is claimed that crying is beneficial for psychological reasons, because they learn that they cannot have immediate satisfaction of impulses. The result is that at two or three months of age (the peak period for crying), some babies spend most of the day and more or less the whole evening – the most common time in the twenty-four hours for babies to cry inconsolably unless picked up and walked around – in a highly distressed state. They only stop crying to fall asleep from exhaustion.[15]

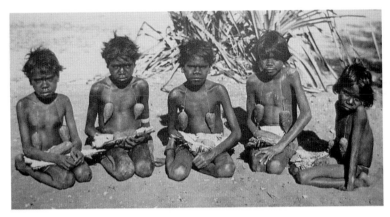

Left: Aboriginal girls play at being mothers, breastfeeding their mud dolls.

Below: A woman in the Philippines successfully combines her work as a farmer and market vendor with breastfeeding her baby.

In Japan mothers never let their babies cry in the first four months of life. They believe that a baby left to cry will develop a habit of crying. Writing about mothers and babies on the island of Okinawa, which was heavily influenced by the US presence after the Second World War, psychologists in the 1960s commented: 'To prevent the formation of this habit, mothers, fathers and grandmothers rush to comfort a crying infant. He is picked up at once, cuddled, nursed, whether he is hungry or not, and if necessary is held for long periods of time until he stops crying.' American health authorities and educators working in Okinawa were obviously having a hard time changing Japanese culture. These writers analysed child rearing practices as typified by 'a lack of enforcing individual achievement striving' and expressed their American value judgements when they wrote of 'extreme indulgence' in baby care.[16]

Breastfeeding

There are striking contrasts in breastfeeding practice and attitudes towards it between traditional cultures and those of industrial societies. Most children in North America and Europe grow up without seeing babies breastfed as a matter of course. Breastfeeding is treated as an intimate and slightly improper act, suited only to the bedroom or bathroom. A woman is expected to be discreet, and if she breastfeeds openly in a public place may be accused of blatant exhibitionism.

In many traditional cultures breastfeeding is a familiar sight. In Australia, Aboriginal girls (and boys, for that matter) learn about breastfeeding because they see it happening around them all the time. It is not a subject for formal learning. Aboriginal girls play at being mothers, but where in industrialised cultures they are given miniature

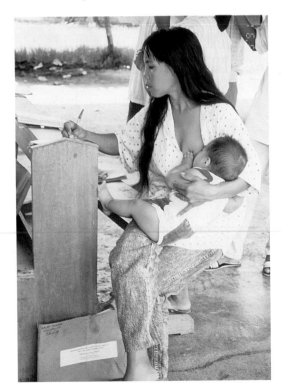

plastic feeding bottles to stick in their dolls' mouths, Aboriginal children's dolls are made of mud and are hung on ropes around their necks so they can feed their babies. An essential part of playing with a doll is the breastfeeding.

In industrial cultures, many children are kept ignorant about breastfeeding. A six-year-old boy who was playing with one of my grandsons noticed my daughter with her baby at the breast, and stood stock still, eyes open wide, and asked if the baby was 'eating' her. I have witnessed a mother remove her eight-year-old daughter from the seat on a train when a woman opposite was breastfeeding her baby.

In the media breastfeeding is marginalised. Content analysis of British TV and press coverage over a period of a month revealed that breastfeeding is rarely shown or discussed.[17] There was only one scene of a breastfeeding baby and 170 scenes of bottles and bottle-feeding. There were forty-two items about breastfeeding difficulties, compared with just one reference to any problem with bottle-feeding.

When breastfeeding is shown on TV it is represented as something done primarily by impoverished women in the Third World, with flies buzzing around them as they struggle to nourish their emaciated babies. Or it is treated as a joke and features embarrassment at the sexuality of exposed breasts. In *Coronation Street*, a barmaid with leaking breasts asks a startled male customer whether he can see that her bra is stuffed with toilet paper. In the American sitcom *Friends*, the baby's father 'freaks out' when a friend tastes breastmilk and says, 'It's gross!' His flatmate remarks, 'But the packaging does appeal to grown-ups!'

It is hardly surprising that new mothers often lack confidence when breastfeeding. Far from being the natural way in which to nurture a baby, producing enough milk and getting it into the baby seems like a complicated conjuring trick which they must practise over and over again, but cannot get right. This is why many women turn to artificial feeding with relief.

In traditional cultures mothers work with their babies cuddled against their bodies. They are rocked, bounced, and often shaken energetically by the movements as they dig and hoe, pound millet, knead bread, scour pots, rub the laundry on stones in the river, or break up rocks to build a road.

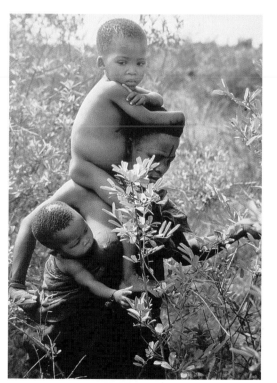

Left: In traditional cultures women work with their babies, who are rocked, bounced and shaken energetically by the movements of their bodies.

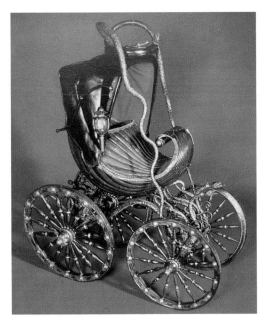

When the sun is high the baby is placed in the shade. An Australian Aboriginal baby sleeps on the ground protected by the basket carrier with which he is attached to his mother's body, and as soon as he stirs he is picked up and fed.

Few women in northern industrial cultures can take their babies to work with them. Our society does not, on the whole, tolerate babies except when they are silent or sleeping. Mothering is perceived as a purely domestic activity.

The roots of intimacy between mother and baby began to be cut in Europe in the 18th century. The process started with the aristocracy. The baby became an object by which social status could be exhibited. A servant could chauffeur the little king in a perambulator, an elaborate conveyance that communicated the family's social standing and wealth. The baby was turned into an indicator of conspicuous consumption.

Peasant mothers and working class women still slept with their babies and breastfed them as a matter of course. So did the rising middle classes, the merchants and teachers, for example, among whom nursing was a family and social occasion. In Flemish paintings, breastfeeding the baby represented the unity, stability and prosperity of the Dutch burgher family.

Above: The earliest known English baby carriage, made for the Duchess of Devonshire's baby in 1730.

Right: Possett-pots, food-warmers and a pewter bottle.

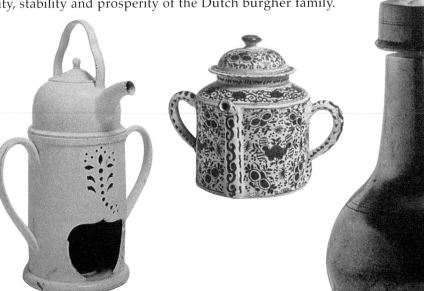

In Italy, the aristocracy sent their babies to wet nurses. It was the husband's responsibility to seek out a healthy peasant woman. If a wet nurse were not available, goats' or cows' milk might be given, often in a pewter bottle which caused lead poisoning. Pap, a mixture of bread and water, was spooned into babies to fatten them up.

In the 19th century middle class women were instructed to breastfeed by male physicians and clerics. There were very strict rules about how they ought to do this. At the turn of the century, for example, an English doctor, Andrew Wilson, published an *Encyclopaedia of Health and Illness* in which he warned that 'infants are very feeble folk, and a nurse must remember how tiny is their frame of life and how swiftly the least chill or carelessness may result in death'.[18] He told mothers that they should put the baby in a separate crib instead of sleeping with it, as most women had done in the past. He stressed the danger of 'over-laying' and said that a woman's 'pendulous breasts may smother a child . . . The little lungs are so small, and hold so little air, that the least thing smothers an infant.' Babies were expected to sleep in isolation and he instructed mothers to 'wash the child's mouth out with boracic lotion after each feeding'.

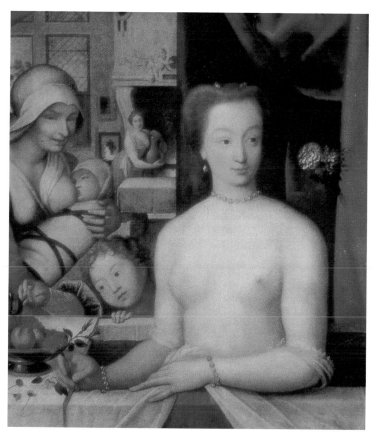

Above: Gabrielle d'Estree with her baby and wet nurse.

Artificial milks were introduced at the beginning of the 20th century. Promotion of formula and other starchy foods to be added to bottles put increasing numbers of babies in danger, since few people knew how to sterilise the equipment, or were able to do so because of the long tubes and corners in which bacteria thrived. The teats were made of chamois leather or were the pickled nipples of calves. With the invention of the vulcanisation of rubber, teats were put on the market which perished with repeated boiling, became bone-hard and had a disgusting odour.

The Industrial Revolution saw women having to leave their homes to work in factories, and this resulted in babies being artificially fed. The *dutty pot* was always sitting on the stove and was a breeding

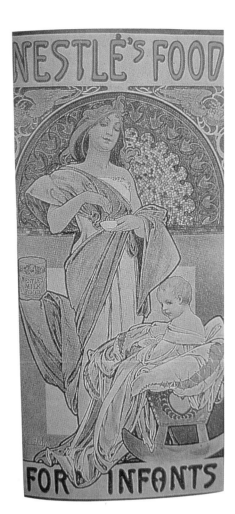

Above: Nestlé was the first company to advertise artificial baby milk and promoted it by telling mothers that they need not be 'like a common cow'.

ground for germs. Babies suffered vitamin deficiency, with resulting rickets. Films promoting artificial milks promised women that their babies would flourish. The very first advertisement for manufactured milk showed a woman who was feeding her baby on formula as a free spirit, and stated that she 'need not condemn herself to be a common "cow" unless she has a real desire to nurse'.

Women who insisted on breastfeeding were sold 'anti-embarrassment devices'. The contraption was patented in 1910 and consisted of a harness which confined the breast, with rubber tubes passing over the breasts, out through the clothing, and ending in artificial nipples for the baby to suck on. A woman who did not wish to breastfeed had her breasts tightly bound with bandages and drank Epsom salts to dry up her milk.

Nurses instructed mothers in how to feed the modern way, using a bottle. But the Mothercraft Movement of the 1920s and 1930s reintroduced breastfeeding. At the same time, it imposed on mothers and babies a military-style discipline. Women were told that they must feed the baby for only two minutes on each side in the days following birth or their nipples would be chewed to shreds. They were allowed to extend this to ten minutes each side, but never longer. They had to stick to rigid schedules and clock-watch feeding sessions. Breastfeeding became a matter for medical advice. There were strict rules about never feeding at night and it was firmly believed by those that gave this advice that babies benefited from prolonged and frantic crying.

Following the Second World War, hospitals were once again fully staffed as doctors returned from the armed services and could take over the organisation of hospitals from nurses and midwives. As a result, newborn babies were isolated from their mothers and lined up in hospital nurseries under the supervision of neonatal nurses and neonatologists.

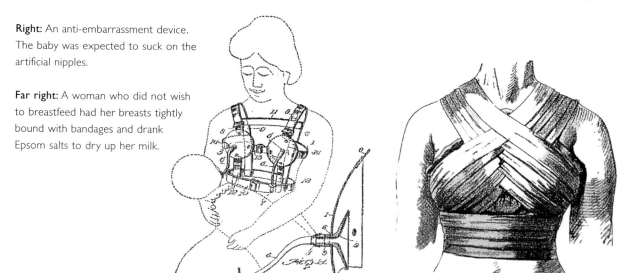

Right: An anti-embarrassment device. The baby was expected to suck on the artificial nipples.

Far right: A woman who did not wish to breastfeed had her breasts tightly bound with bandages and drank Epsom salts to dry up her milk.

It was a paediatrician, Doctor Benjamin Spock, who introduced the concept of breastfeeding on demand; this soon began to replace the rigid feeding schedules. It had become obvious that many babies were unhappy or failed to thrive when mothers fed by the clock. Spock's teaching advised mothers to get to know their babies and respond to their needs.

Yet even women who feed on demand often lack confidence in baby-led breastfeeding, and many still seek guidance from professionals. Those who take professional advice feed their babies less often than women who simply get on with it. Throughout Europe there is wide variation in practice among mothers who say they are feeding on demand. In Germany this means an average of 5.7 feeds a day, in Portugal 8.5 feeds a day, and in Spain mothers feed two-month-old babies 7 times a day.[19] Commenting on this, 'Minerva' writes in the *British Medical Journal*: 'Perhaps midwives, general practitioners, and obstetricians are bigger fans of scheduled feeding than they let on.'[20]

Birth does not end with the delivery of a baby. It is part of a continuum that develops into the relationship between a mother and her baby at the breast. Breastfeeding is not only a method of getting milk into a baby. It is a way of loving. Their relationship grows out of the interdependence that existed between the mother and baby while the child was still inside her body. But because the baby is no longer in her uterus it is possible to fragment it, even to destroy it utterly, by choice, by accident, or because a child-rearing culture forces a woman to break the intimacy of that relationship.

Out of the interdependence between a mother and her baby a child's independence grows. From this closeness comes a child's ability to move out with confidence into the world.

Chapter 9

Can We Learn Anything From Other Cultures?

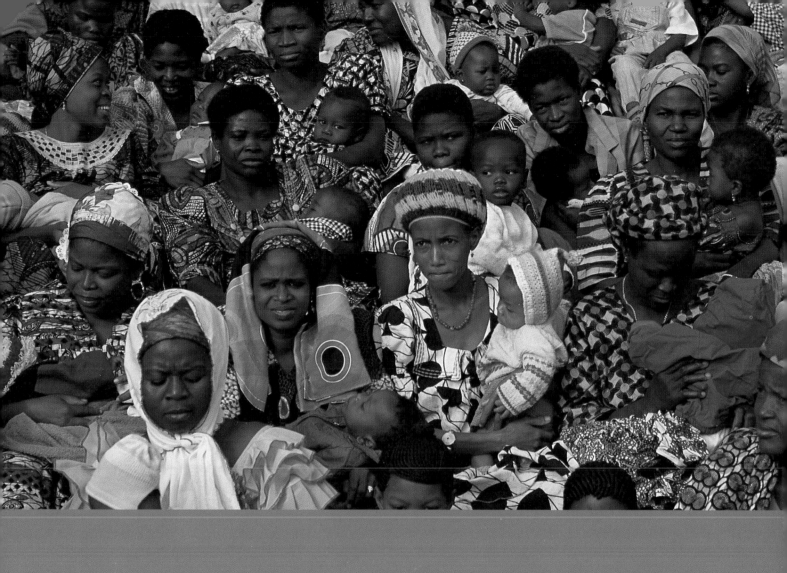

As we have explored traditional ways of birth through these pages, a contrast between the social and technocratic models of childbirth has emerged.

According to the technocratic model typical of North America and Europe today, birth is a potentially pathological process, and only 'normal' in retrospect. Labour and delivery are the work of an obstetric team rather than the woman herself. Each pregnant woman is evaluated in terms of risk categories, and from early pregnancy onwards she is turned into a patient, the object of medical care, concern and screening. There is often little continuity of care and a large number of different, and often anonymous specialists may be involved. Emotional and spiritual aspects of birth are usually ignored or treated as embarrassing.

The social model, in contrast, defines birth as a social event and normal life process. It entails hard work that is done by the woman, her close family, female friends and other women in the neighbourhood, including a midwife who is well-known in the community. Her helpers are almost exclusively women. She has continuity of care and a continuing relationship with those who provide the care. The mother is seen as passing through a major life transition in which spiritual forces must be invoked to support her, and evil spirits and negative psychological influences kept at bay. Emotional and spiritual aspects of birth are central to the experience of everyone participating.

The technocratic model requires women to be removed from their normal environment of the home, in which they are in control, and to go to a hospital to give birth. It is alien territory, a setting usually associated with sickness, injury and death, and it is often a great distance from the mother's home. Everything the woman does – her behaviour, her movements and the sounds she is allowed to make – is controlled and restricted by the hospital environment.

In the social model the woman gives birth at home or in her mother's home, in a birth hut or enclosure that her husband has built for her, in the familiar territory of the hut which women share when they are menstruating, or in the women's bath house.

Within the technocratic model the mother is attended by male and female strangers who may not have given birth themselves. They are professionals with esoteric knowledge that is not shared with her. They use a language distinct from ordinary, everyday language and communicate with each other about this without the mother being able to understand what is being said. The relationship between professional care-givers and patients, though it can be friendly and emotionally supportive, is basically one of dominance and subordination.

In the social model of childbirth the mother is attended by older women who are mothers themselves. Knowledge and decision-making is shared. Familiar language and imagery is used and there is an equal relationship between care-givers and the woman giving birth.

The elimination of pain by powerful and effective anaesthesia, or its reduction by analgesia, distinguishes the technocratic from the social model of childbirth and makes other interventions possible. Caesarean section is practical only when a woman can be promised anaesthesia. In social childbirth women know that they have to handle pain, and do not expect birth to be painless.

The techniques used in the two models of childbirth are very different. According to a technocratic model, birth is typified by routine obstetric intervention. During their professional training obstetricians acquire highly sophisticated technical skills, assisted by electronic apparatus to handle complicated and obstructed labours with uterine stimulation, intravenous fluids and surgery.

In contrast, in social childbirth interventions are few and far between. Care-givers have a range of comfort skills, including massage, hot and cold compresses, holding the labouring woman and using verbal and visual imagery for its psychological effect. In most traditional cultures the midwife does not perform vaginal examinations or give injections unless she has been influenced by the prevailing medical model of birth and believes that this is something that ought to be done. Any interventions tend to be non-invasive. There are, however, few resources with which to handle complicated or obstructed labour. When a baby is not lying in a good position, the head is too large to pass through a pelvis which has been misshapen by malnutrition in childhood, the placenta does not separate completely in the third stage and the mother haemorrhages, or when the cord is cut with a dirty knife, resulting in sepsis, birth is much more dangerous for both mother and baby.

Time is perceived differently in the technocratic and social models of birth. Medical management entails framing and measuring time in small segments. The progress of birth is assessed in terms of the clock. With the care system known as 'active management', women are guaranteed a labour that will not be allowed to last longer than twelve hours, though this is likely to mean that the uterus must be artificially stimulated. If the uterus fails to respond with increased efficiency, or the drugs employed have a negative effect on the fetus, delivery must be completed by Caesarean section.

In social childbirth time is related to natural phenomena, such as sunrise and sunset, and the progress of birth is assessed in social terms: the coming and going of different people, and regular household events such as meals or taking goats to pasture. If the uterus is working well this may be reassuring. But labour may continue for days, sometimes causing the mother great distress and harming the baby.

A woman who has a baby in hospital is usually put to bed. Even when she is allowed or encouraged to walk around, the bed is often centrally placed in the room. The only place in which to walk may be a corridor, the only place to sit comfortably the television room. She has a passive role, at least until her cervix is declared fully dilated. At that point she is urged to strain and push for as long and as hard as she can, often in a reclining position or flat on her back with her legs in lithotomy stirrups.

With the social model of childbirth, labour is perceived as activity. The woman is not expected to lie on a bed, and, indeed, there may be no bed in the room, and certainly no delivery table. She uses ordinary household objects such as a rope, a stool, a hammock, a chair or a house post to give her support. She finds different positions that feel right for her and the baby at that time, often at the suggestion of the midwife, who combines these postural changes with massage to ease pain and to rotate the baby. Birth becomes like a dance in which the other women present join with the labouring woman to rock, rotate and tilt the pelvis, and to give her physical support as she moves. She is usually in an upright or semi-upright position as she pushes the baby out, squatting, kneeling, half-squatting, half-kneeling, standing or on all fours.

When the baby is about to be delivered, the woman whose birth is being managed medically is likely to have an episiotomy. In some countries the obstetrician may hook a finger or thumb in her anus to push the baby's chin forward and expedite delivery, too. Once the head is on the perineum the baby is got out at top speed. The mother is stitched up afterwards.

With the social model of birth, the time from the appearance of the baby's head on the perineum to the birth may be prolonged. If the head is a tight fit or there is malpresentation this is likely to be very hard on the mother's perineal tissues, and she may have a tear from the vagina into the rectum. In cultures in which there is no possibility of perineal repair she may be left with a vesico-vaginal fistula, incontinent and passing faeces through her vagina. This may make her an outcast.

With the technocratic model of childbirth, active management of the third stage entails immediate clamping and cutting of the cord and the injection of an oxytocic drug to empty the uterus. In certain countries the obstetrician pulls the cervix down with forceps in order to inspect it for damage and sweeps a hand round inside the uterus to ensure that there are no 'retained products'.

A woman escapes these very painful interventions in the social model characteristic of traditional cultures, but there may be little that can be done if she bleeds heavily, and sometimes she bleeds to death.

The delivery of the placenta is managed conservatively in social childbirth. Unless the midwife has come into contact with Western obstetrics, she is wary of pulling on the cord, and may get the mother to cough, give her something that makes her sneeze or vomit, or have her blow into a bottle or a hollow gourd. Or she may administer oxytocic herbs to stimulate uterine activity.

Today, few of us who live in industrialised cultures would choose a social model of childbirth in which there was no possibility of obstetric intervention even though it might be life-saving. But many women would like birth to take place without drugs or surgery, in an environment in which their bodies have a chance to work spontaneously and which they themselves can control.

But, because birth practices are rooted in culture, and are part of a co-ordinated and interdependent system of beliefs about reproduction, women, life and death, it is difficult to pick and choose elements from traditional birth cultures and transfer them to a technocratic birth culture without changing them in the process. These changes may be beneficial, but we need to be aware of what we are doing, and must also realise that such practices, suitably modified, can be incorporated into a hospital system so as to provide attractive options for women who might otherwise decide on a home birth.

It is equally difficult to introduce practices from the technocratic model into a traditional birth culture without changing that culture in unanticipated ways. When plastic sheets and fertiliser bags are used for delivery, oxytocin is injected routinely in order to stimulate the uterus, and a dirty knife is used to cut the cord instead of a fresh sliver of bamboo, or when babies are fed on artificial milk from unsterilised bottles and teats rather than being put to the breast, 'modern' practices bring new dangers.

There are sound reasons, validated by research, why a woman may prefer to avoid regular ultrasound examinations, continuous electronic fetal monitoring in labour and routine episiotomy at delivery. But it is rarely easy to ensure that she does not receive these interventions. She may meet outright opposition, be told that what she is asking for risks her baby's life, or, at best, encounter amused condescension.

It is easier to introduce practices from the technocratic model of birth into a traditional culture than to introduce traditional practices into the system of medical management. This is partly because medical practice is backed by international firms that manufacture and promote the drugs, electronics and surgical instruments used. At every medical conference, and many conferences of midwives, childbirth educators and consumer organisations, there is an exhibition hall filled with such products. There are huge profits to be made by exporting these things to developing countries. There is no money to be made from a rope hanging from the rafters or a birth stool. The aggressive marketing of medical technology includes sponsorship of conferences, research projects, trips overseas, provision of free equipment and other 'gifts', and glossy literature.

When high technology takes over in poor countries it is a dangerous substitute for low technology projects that have a major positive impact on health, and it tends to eat up the health care budget. Access to clean water saves more lives than ultrasound in doctors' offices, electronic fetal monitors in the delivery room and incubators in an intensive care nursery.

Birth is a political issue, not just a matter of individual preference. Birth options are sometimes discussed as if they were similar to selecting brands of cereal or cans of beans on a supermarket shelf. You take the most attractive on offer. Yet the birth choices we make affect women in other parts of the world. If an epidural or an elective Caesarean is seen as providing the best kind of birth, these quickly become the goal everywhere for those who can afford private obstetrics. Eventually they may be the norm for all births, if only because doctors do not know how to deliver babies in any other way.

What is happening in childbirth today is similar to the change from breast- to bottle-feeding that occurred in the first half of the 20th century. Middle class women, many of them following doctors' advice, came to believe that artificial feeding was more reliable and convenient than breastfeeding, more and more women had difficulty establishing breastfeeding, and infant formula manufacturers expanded rapidly to meet a ready market. Now, when middle class women hope to once again breastfeed, poorer women in our own societies and those in developing parts of the world have been taught to believe that artificial baby milk is as good as, or better than, human milk. They are told that if they want to do the best they can for their babies they should pay for a product which formula manufacturers promote as a substitute milk 'when breastfeeding fails', and as a complementary and 'follow-on' milk. The direct result is that babies are unable to resist infection, and suffer from gastro-enteritis and other diseases because they are not breastfed.

When a pregnant woman makes choices about birth it may seem too demanding to expect her to think of our culture of birth also in political and economic terms. It is hard enough to get the information she needs and to examine the research evidence in order to make decisions. Even when she has that information, it is often difficult to negotiate what she wants. When she makes a birth plan and discusses it with her care-givers she may come to feel that they are treating her as over-anxious, ungrateful and 'difficult'. It is very easy to be put down, and she may fear that if she continues to struggle for the kind of birth she wants she will be penalised for it or her baby will suffer. It is important for women to join together to explore the issues surrounding birth and not let them be treated only as a personal matter.

This is a challenge for all of us, nationally and internationally, not only for our own sakes, but for our daughters, and their daughters after them. If, through fear or ignorance, we neglect our heritage and allow technocracy to take over, woman-centred childbirth may be lost forever.

At Sheila Kitzinger's web site: **www.sheilakitzinger.com**

you can explore various aspects of birth, drawing on things that Sheila has learned from women around the world and her research as a social anthropologist into women's experiences of pregnancy, birth and breastfeeding. Get up-to-date information about midwifery, home birth and waterbirth. Link to articles referred to in this book that are available on the Internet, and to web pages of useful organisations.

Footnotes

Introduction

1 Scully D., Men Who Control Women's Health, Houghton Mifflin, Boston, 1980
2 Lomas, M., Enkin, M., et al, 'Opinion leader vs audit and feedback to implement practice guidelines', Journal of American Medical Association, 265, 1991, pp2202-7
3 Davis-Floyd, R., Birth as an American Rite of Passage, University of California Press, Berkeley, 1992

Chapter 1

1 Scheper-Hughes, N., 'Virgin Mothers: The Impact of Irish Jansenism on Childbearing and Infant Tending in Western Ireland' in Kay, M. A., Anthropology of Human Birth, F A Davis, Philadelphia, 1982, p277
2 Hahn, R. A. & Muecke, M. A., Current Problems in Obstetrics, Gynecology and Fertility: The Anthropology of Birth in Five US Ethnic Populations, Yearbook Medical Publishers, Chicago, 1987, pp154-157
3 Chamberlain, D. B., 'Babies Are Not What We Thought - Call for a New Paradigm', International Journal of Prenatal and Perinatal Studies, Vol. 4, 314, 1992, pp1-17
4 Macfarlane, A., The Family Life of Ralph Josselin 1616-1683, Cambridge University Press, 1976
5 Newman, K., Fetal Positions: Individualism, Science, Visuality, Stanford University Press, Stanford, 1996, pp69-82
6 Fraser, R. & Watson, R., 'Bleeding during the latter half of pregnancy' in Chalmers, I., Enkin, M., Keirse, M. J. N. C. (eds), Effective Care in Pregnancy and Childbirth, Vol. 1, Oxford University Press, 1989, pp594-611
7 Brand, I. R., Kaminopetros, P., Cave, M., et al, 'Specificity of antenatal ultrasound in the Yorkshire region: a prospective study of 2261 ultrasound detected anomalies', British Journal of Obstetrics and Gynaecology, Vol. 101, 5, 1994, pp392-397
8 Berger, A., Science Editor, British Medical Journal, 318, 1999, p85
9 Saari-Kemppainen, A., Karjalainen, L., Ylosalo, P., et al, 'Ultrasound screening and perinatal mortality: controlled trial of systematic one-stage screening in pregnancy. The Helsinki ultrasound trial', Lancet, Vol. 336, 8712, 1990, pp387-391, and Newnham, J. P., Evans, S. F., Michael, C. A., et al, 'Effects of frequent ultrasound during pregnancy: a randomised controlled trial', Lancet, Vol. 342, 8876, 1993, pp887-891
10 Kishwar, M., 'When daughters are unwanted', Manushi 86, January/February 1995, quoted in Newsletter of Birth Traditions Survival Bank, Department of Midwifery, University of Central Lancashire, Preston, Vol. 4, 3, 1995, pp14-16,
11 Khanna Sunil, K., 'Prenatal sex determination: a new family building strategy', Manushi 86, January/February 1995, quoted in Newsletter of Birth Traditions Survival Bank, op.cit., pp11-14
12 Khanna Sunil, K., op. cit.
13 Kishwar, M., op. cit.
14 Daikanwa Jiten Showa 61, (3rd ed) Vol. 13, p9628, Showa 33 (1st ed), Tokyo: Taishukan
15 Nihon Kokuga Daijiten, Showa 49, Vol. 12, p529, Tokyo: Shogakkan
16 Stucken, E., Astralmythen, p119, Leipzig: Eduard Pfeiffer, 1907
17 Morsy, S., 'Childbirth in an Egyptian Village' in Kay, M. A., op. cit., p159
18 Author's field research in Jamaica
19 Cressy, D., Birth, Marriage & Death: ritual, religion, and the life-cycle in Tudor and Stuart England, Oxford University Press, 1997, p45
20 Smith, F. B., The People's Health 1830-1910, Croom Helm, London, 1979, p15
21 DeLee, J., Obstetrics for Nurses, W B Saunders, Philadelphia, 1904, pp78-79
22 Barker, D. J. P. (ed) 'Fetal and infant origins of adult disease', BMJ Publishing Group, London, 1992
23 Nathanielsz, P., Life in the Womb: The Origin of Health and Disease, Promethean Press, New York, 1999
24 Ianniruberto, A. & Tajani, E., 'Ultra sonographic study of fetal movements', Seminars in Peri-natology 5, 1981, pp175-181
25 Chamberlain, D. B., op. cit.
26 Chamberlain, D. B., op. cit.

Chapter 2

1 Kavasch, E. B. & Barr, K., American Indian Healing Arts, Thorson, London, 1999, p136
2 Mitchell, F., quoted in Kavasch & Barr, op. cit., p135
3 Kitzinger, S., Ourselves as Mothers, Bantam, London, 1993, p130
4 Kitzinger, S., A Celebration of Birth, Penny Press, 1986. ICEA PO Box 20048, Minneapolis, Minnesota 55420, USA. Fax: 612/854-87721
5 Randolph, V., Ozark Superstitions, Columbia University Press, New York, 1947
6 Chohoki, O., A Useful Reference Book for Women, Tokyo National Diet Library, 1692
7 Cassidy, C. M., Subcultural Prenatal Diets of Americans in Alternative Dietary Practices and Nutritional Abuses in Pregnancy, National Academy Press, Washington DC, 1982, pp25-60
8 Chohoki, O., op. cit.
9 Cosminsky, S., 'Childbirth and Change: A Guatemalan Study' in MacCormick, C. P. (ed) Ethnography of Fertility and Birth, Academic Press, London and New York, 1982, pp205-229
10 Cosminsky, S., op. cit.
11 Laderman, C., Wives and Midwives: Childbirth and Nutrition in Rural Malaysia, University of California Press, Berkeley, 1983
12 Januke, S., 'When The Mother-To-Be Drinks', Childbirth Instructor, Winter 1994, pp28-35
13 Gerarde, J., 'The Berball or Generall Historie of Plantes', 1636, quoted in Cressy, op. cit., p47
14 Sharp, J., Midwives Book, pp181-2, 206-10; Culpeper, Directory for Midwives, p150, quoted in David Cressy, op. cit., p47
15 Mathews, F., Yudkin, P. & Neil, A., 'Folates in the periconceptual period: are women getting enough?', British Journal of Obstetrics and Gynaecology, 105, 1998, pp954-959
16 Alberman, E., & Noble, J. M., 'Commentary: Food should be fortified with folic acid', British Medical Journal, 319, 1999, p93
17 Cosminsky, S., op. cit., pp205-229
18 Author's interview with Dr Yoshimura

19 Ballantyne, J. W., The Byrth of Mankynd (its Authors and Editions), reprints from Journal of Obstetrics and Gynaecology of the British Empire, 1906
20 Brady, M. Y., Having A Baby Easily, Health For All Publishing Company, London, 1944, pp59-60 (first published as Natural Childbirth, Heinemann, London, 1933)
21 Dick-Read, G., Childbirth Without Fear, Heinemann, London, 1972, pp56-59
22 Mahoney, T. & Slone, L., The Grape Merchants, Harper and Rowe, New York, 1966, p249
23 Heller, Z., Sunday Times, 13 December 1998
24 Mills, Y., Sunday Times Style, 20 December 1998
25 Clement, S., 'Childbirth on Television', British Journal of Midwifery, 5, 1, 1997, pp37-42
26 Cobb, J., 'Birth on the Box', New Generation, December 1995, pp3-4
27 Handfield, B., 'Lights, Camera, Action . . . Childbirth!', Pregnancy, Spring 1998, pp58-60
28 Channel 4 TV, London
29 Watts, G., 'Science, Sense and Substance', British Medical Journal, Vol. 317, 1998, p1462
30 Diepenbrock, C., ' "God willed it!" Gynecology at the check-out stand: reproductive technology in the women's service magazine, 1977-1996' in Gavron, C., Gurak, L. J., Lay, M. M. & Myutti, C., Body Talk: Rhetoric, Technology and Reproduction, University of Wisconsin Press, Madison, 2000
31 Diepenbrock, C., op. cit.
32 Patients' Guide to IVF Clinics, London, 1998
33 Connor, S., The Independent, 28 December 1998
34 Selye, H., The Stress of Life, McGraw-Hill, New York, 1976

Chapter 3

1 Stone, M., Ancient Mirrors of Womanhood Vol. 2, New Sibylline Books, New York, 1980, p64 adapted
2 Stone, M., op. cit., p92 adapted
3 Waley, A., The Way and its Power, Allen and Unwin, London, 1934, p149
4 Stone, M., op. cit., p37 adapted
5 Adapted from Campbell, J., Occidental Mythology, The Masks of God Vol. III, Secker and Warburg, London, 1965
6 Allen, M., The Birth Symbol in Traditional Women's Art from Eurasia and the Western Pacific, Toronto Museum for Textiles catalogue, 1981, p29
7 Campbell, J. op cit., adapted
8 Allen, M., op. cit., p26
9 Stone, M., op. cit., p78 adapted
10 Stone, M., op. cit., pp1-4 adapted
11 Stone, M., op. cit., p27 adapted
12 Stone, M., op. cit., p167 adapted
13 Stone, M., op. cit., p76
14 Homer, Odyssey, Vol. 1
15 Stone, M., op. cit., p64 adapted
16 Kitzinger, S., A Celebration of Birth, op. cit.
17 Larrington, C. (ed.) The Feminist Companion to Mythology, Parelara, London, 1992, pp102-117
18 Knipe, R., The Water of Life: A Jungian Journey through Hawaiian Myth, University of Hawaii Press, Honolulu, 1989, p32
19 Henderson, H. K. & Henderson, R. N., 'Traditional Onitsha Ibo maternity beliefs and practices' in Kay, M. A., op. cit.

20 Laderman, C., 'Giving birth in a Malay village' in Kay, M. A., op. cit.
21 Eiseman Jnr, F. B., Bali: Sekala and Niskala Vol. 1: Essays on Religion, Ritual, and Arts, Periplus Editions, Berkeley, 1989, pp85, 90
22 Recio, D. M., 'Birth and Tradition in the Philippines' in Maglaos (ed.) The Potential of the Traditional Birth Attendant, WHO, 1986
23 Skeat, W. W., Malay Magic, Oxford University Press, 1899, 1984
24 Chawla, J., Child Bearing and Culture - Woman Centered Revisioning of the Traditional Midwife: the Dai as a Ritual Practitioner, Indian Social Institute, New Delhi, 1994
25 Quoted in Cressy, D., op. cit., p.65
26 Dévotions particulières pour les femmes enceintes, p21, Paris 1665
27 Biesele, M., 'An Ideal of Unassisted Birth' in Davis-Floyd, R. E. & Sargent, C. F. (eds), Childbirth and Authoritative Knowledge, University of California Press, Berkeley, 1997, p.485
28 Cressy, D., op. cit., pp16-17
29 Cressy, D., op. cit., pp20-21
30 Cressy, D., op. cit., p21
31 Cressy, D., op. cit., p23
32 Forbes, T. R., The Midwife and the Witch, Yale University Press, New Haven, 1966
33 Forbes, T. R., op. cit.
34 Wertz, R. W. & D. C., Lying-In: A History of Childbirth in America, Free Press, New York, 1977, p23
35 Ulrich, L. T., Good Wives, Image and Reality in the Lives of Women in Northern New England 1650-1750, Vintage Press, New York, 1991, p129
36 Wertz, R. W. & D. C., op. cit., pp25-26
37 Radio Times, 31 October 1998
38 Milton, G. in Chester, P. (ed.) Sisters on a Journey: Portraits of American Midwives, Rutgers University Press, New Brunswick, 1997, pp193-4
39 Kahn, R. P., Bearing meaning: the language of birth, University of Illinois Press, Chicago, 1995
40 Chester, P. (ed.), op. cit., p170
41 Munroe, S. in Chester, P. (ed.), op. cit., p197
42 Murdaugh, Sister A. in Chester, P. (ed.), op. cit., p200
43 Gibson, F. in Chester, P. (ed.), op. cit., p147
44 Gaskin, I. M., Spiritual Midwifery, Paul Mandelstein, Summerton, Ten., 1978
45 Luthy, D. A., Shy, K. K., van Belle, G. et al, 'A Randomized Trial of Electronic Fetal Monitoring in Preterm Labor.', Journal of Obstetrics and Gynecology, Vol. 69, 5, 1987, pp687-695; MacDonald, D., Grant, A., Sheridan-Pereira, M. et al, 'The Dublin Randomized Controlled Trial of Intrapartum Fetal Heart Rate Monitoring' Journal of Obstetrics and Gynecology, Vol. 152, 5, 1985, pp524-539

Chapter 4

1 Odent, M., The Scientification of Love, Free Association Books, London, 1999, p23
2 Odent, M., op. cit., p21
3 Odent, M., op. cit., p22
4 Konner, M. in Eaton, S. B., Shostak, M. & Konner, M., The Paleolithic Prescription: A program of diet and exercises and a design for living, Harper and Rowe, New York, 1988, quoted in Odent, M., op. cit., p23
5 Biesele, M., 'An Ideal of Unassisted Birth' in Davis-Floyd, R. E. & Sargent, C. F. (eds), op. cit., p474
6 Sargent, C., 'Solitary Confinement: Birth Practices Among the Bariba of the People's Republic of Benin' in Kay, M. A., op. cit.
7 Bourque, S. C. & Warre, K. B., Women of the Andes: Patriarchy and Social Change in Two Peruvian Towns, University of Michigan Press, Ann Arbor, 1981
8 Awang Hasmadi Aswang Mois, 'Beliefs and practices concerning births among the Selako of Sarawak', Sarawak Museum Journal, Vol. xxvi, 47, 1978, pp7-13
9 Hundt, G., Ph.D. thesis, University of Warwick
10 Mezey, G. C., 'Domestic violence in pregnancy' in Bewley, S., Friend, J., & Mezey, G. (eds) Violence Against Women, RCOG Press, London, 1997, pp191-198
11 Elliot, J. K., The Apocryphal New Testament, Clarendon Press, Oxford, 1993, p93
12 Cressy, D., op. cit., pp56-58
13 Cressy, D., op. cit., pp56-58
14 Cressy, D., op. cit., pp56-58
15 Cressy, D., op. cit., p85
16 Hill, R., The Pathway to Prayer and Pietie, 1610, quoted in Cressy, D., op. cit., p85
17 Cited in Leavitt, J. W., Brought To Bed: Child-Bearing in America 1750-1950, Oxford University Press, p37
18 Cited in Leavitt, J. W., op. cit., p37
19 Leavitt, J. W., op. cit., pp96-97
20 The Diary of Samuel Sewall, 1674-1729, Collections of the Massachusetts Historical Society, p394
21 Anita McCormick Blaine to Lettie Fowler McCormick, August 1890, McCormick papers, Wisconsin State Historical Society archives, quoted in Leavitt, J. W., op. cit., p89
22 McCall, D. L., The Copper King's Daughter: From Cape Cod to Crooked River, Binfords and Mort, Portland, Oregon, 1972
23 Quoted in Cooper, P. & Buford, N. B., The Quilters Women and Domestic Art, Anchor Press/Doubleday, New York, 1978, p15
24 Landrum, S. H., Letter to editor, Journal of American Medical Association, p576, 1912, quoted in Leavitt, J. W., op. cit., p61
25 Wertz, R. W. & D. C., op. cit., p73
26 Anon., Medical Knowledge, The Works of the Famous Philosopher, J. Smith, London, date unknown
27 Loudon, I., 'Obstetrics and the general practitioner', British Medical Journal, Vol. 301, 1990, pp705-7
28 Loudon, I., Western Medicine, Oxford University Press, 1997, p217
29 Loudon, I., 'Obstetric care, social class and maternal mortality', British Medical Journal, Vol. 293, 1986, pp606-608
30 Loudon, I., Death in Childbirth, Clarendon Press, Oxford, 1992, p251
31 Allison, J., Delivered At Home, Chapman and Hall, London, 1996, p24
32 Allison, J., op. cit., pp79-80
33 Allison, J., op. cit., p84
34 Bourne, G., Pregnancy, Pan, London, 1975
35 Morsy, S. A., 'Childbirth in an Egyptian Village' in Kay, M. A., op. cit., pp147-174
36 Moser, M. B., 'Seri: From Conception through Infancy' in Kay, M. A., op. cit., pp221-232
37 Maggie Akerolik quoted in Special Report on Traditional Midwifery, Suvaguuq, X, 1, Pauktuutit, Inuit Women's Association of Canada, Ottawa 1995
38 Betty Peryouar quoted in Suvaguuq, op. cit.
39 Mary Tagoona quoted in Suvaguuq, op. cit.
40 Personal communication, obstetrician in Osaka
41 van Daalen, R., 'Family Change and Continuity in the Netherlands: Birth and Childbed in Text and Art' in Abraham-Van der Mark, E. (ed.), Successful Home Birth and Midwifery : The Dutch Model, Het Spinhuis, Amsterdam, 1996, p77
42 Katz Rothman, B., 'Going Dutch: Lessons for Americans' in Abraham-Van der Mark, E. (ed.) op. cit., p208
43 Hodnett, E. D., 'Support from caregivers during childbirth' in Enkin, M. W., Keirse, M. J. N. C., Renfrew, M. J., Neilson, J. P. (eds) Pregnancy and Childbirth Module of Cochrane Database of Systematic Reviews, 1995 (updated 24 February 1995). BMJ: London
44 Hodnett E. D., 'Support from caregivers during childbirth', op. cit.
45 Sosa, R., Kennell, J., Klaus, M. et al, 'The effect of a supportive companion on perinatal problems, length of labor and mother-infant interaction', New England Journal of Medicine, Vol. 305, 11, 1980, pp585-7
46 Kennell, J., Klaus, M., McGrath, S. et al, 'Continuous emotional support during labor in a US hospital: a randomised controlled trial', Journal of American Medical Association, Vol. 265, 17, 1991, pp2197-2201
47 Bréart, G., Mlika-Cabane, N., Kaminski, M. et al, 'Evaluation of different policies for the management of labour', Early Human Development, Vol. 29, 1992, pp309-312
48 Hofmeyr, G. J., Nikodem, V. C., Wolman, W. L. et al, 'Companionship to modify the clinical birth environment: effects on progress and perceptions of labour and breastfeeding', British Journal of Obstetrics and Gynaecology, Vol. 98, 8, 1991, pp756-764
49 Hodnett, E. D. & Osborn, R. W., 'A randomised trial of the effects of monitrice support during labor: mothers' views two to four weeks postpartum', Birth 16 (4), 1989, pp177-183
50 Hofmeyr, G. J., Nikodem, V. C., Wolman, W. L et al, op. cit.
51 Kennell, J., Klaus, M., McGrath, S. et al, op. cit.
52 Hofmeyr, G. J., Nikodem, V. C., Wolman, W. L. et al, op. cit.
53 Banyana Madi, C., 'The effects of social support in labour' in The Art and Science of Midwifery, Proceedings of the International Confederation of Midwives, Oslo, 1996, pp267-70
54 Bertsch, T. D., Nagashima-Whalen, L., Dykeman, L. et al, 'Labor support by first-time fathers', Journal of Psychosomatic Obstetrics and Gynecology, 11, 1990, pp251-60
55 Klaus, M. H., Kennell, J. H., & Klaus, P. H., op cit.
56 From the author's own discussion groups with midwives

Chapter 5

1 King, H., 'Bound to bleed: Artemis and Greek women' in Cameron, A. & Kuht, A. (eds) Images of Women in Antiquity, Croom Helm, London, 1983

2 Chryssanthopoulou, V., An Analysis of Rituals Surrounding Birth in Modern Greece, M. Phil. thesis, Bodleian Library, Oxford, 1984

3 Klein, M., Be Fruitful and Multiply, Jerusalem: Museum of the Diaspora, 1987

4 McGilvray, D., 'Sexual power and fertility in Sri Lanka: Matticaloa Tamils and Moors' in McCormack, C. (ed) Ethnography of Fertility and Childbirth, Academic Press, London/New York, 1982

5 Knocki, F., Navajo traditional midwife, personal communication

6 Rayhald, T., The Byrth of Mankyinde, London, 1545

7 McDonald, W. & Davis, J. A., History of Midwifery Practice in Australia and the Western Pacific Regions, Twentieth Congress International Confederation of Midwives, Sydney, 1984, pp23-25, p45

8 Margaret Charles Smith quoted in Holmes, L. J., Listen to Me Good; The Life Story of an Alabama Midwife, Ohio State University Press, Columbus, 1996, p87

9 Margaret Charles Smith quoted in Holmes, L. J., op. cit., pp147-148

10 Speert, H., 'Midwives, Nurses, and Nurse-midwives' in Obstetrics and Gynecology in America: a History, American College of Obstetricians and Gynecologists, Chicago, 1980

11 Anon., in Wertz, R. W. & D. C., op. cit., p57

12 Storer, H., 'Criminal Abortion' in Wertz, R. W. & D. C., op. cit., p57

13 Pence Rooks, J., Midwifery and Childbirth in America, Temple University Press, Philadelphia, 1997, pp21-22

14 G. L. Meigs quoted in Pence Rooks, J., op. cit., p23

15 Williams, J. W., 'Medical Education and the Midwife Problem in the United States', Journal of American Medical Association, 2, 1912, pp180-204

16 Devitt, N., 'The Statistical case for Elimination of the Midwife: Fact versus Prejudice, 1890-1955', Women and Health 4 (1), 1979, pp 81-96; 4 (2) pp169-183. Quoted in Pence Rooks, J., op. cit., p29

17 Devitt, N., in Pence Rooks, J., op. cit., p30

18 Thom, S., in Pence Rooks, J., op. cit., p3

19 Margaret Charles Smith quoted in Holmes, L. J, op. cit., p65

20 Margaret Charles Smith quoted in Holmes, L. J., op. cit., p66

21 Allison, J., Delivered at Home, Chapman and Hall, London, 1996, p85

22 Allison, J., op. cit., p82

23 Hird, C., & Burtch, B., 'Midwives and Safe Motherhood: International Perspectives' in Shroff, F. M., The New Midwifery: Reflections on Renaissance and Regulation, Women's Press, Toronto, 1977, pp115-145

24 Ulrich, L. T., The Midwife's Tale: The Life of Martha Ballard, p189

25 Vincent, P., Department of Midwifery, University of Central Lancashire, Preston, PR1 2HE, Lancs.

26 Botha, M. C., 'The Management of the Umbilical Cord in Labour', South African Journal of Obstetrics and Gynaecology, 24 August 1968, pp30-33

27 The Prevention and Management of Postpartum Haemorrhage, Report of a Technical Working Group, 1989, WHO, Geneva, 1990

28 Fischer, A., 'Reproduction in Truk', Ethnology, Vol.12, 1963, pp526-540

29 Annual Review of Bureau of American Ethnology 1885-1886, Government Printing Office, Washington DC, 1891

30 Recio, D. M., 'Birth and Tradition in the Philippines', in Maglaos (ed.), The Potential of the Traditional Birth Attendant, WHO, Geneva, 1986

31 Coxe Stevenson, M., The Zuni Indians, 23rd Report of US Bureau of American Ethnology, 1905

32 Bridges, L. & Guede, N., No More For Ever: a Saharan Jewish Town, Papers of Peabody Museum of Archeology and Ethnology, Vol. 31. Cambridge Mass., 1947; Schwab, G., Tribes of the Liberian Hinterland, Papers of Peabody Museum, op. cit.

33 Hrdliska, A., Physiological and Medical Observations among the Indians of the South Western United States and Northern Mexico, Bulletin 34, Smithsonian Institution and Bureau of American Ethnology, 1908

34 Engelmann, G., Labour Among Primitive Peoples, p110

35 Sudan Department of Statistics

36 Boddy, J., 'Remembering Amal-birth in Northern Sudan' in Lock, M. & Kaufert, P. A. (eds), Pragmatic Women and Body Politics, Cambridge University Press, 1998, pp40-41

37 Boddy, J., op. cit., pp47-48

38 Quoted in Graham, I. D., Episiotomy: Challenging Obstetric Interventions, Blackwell Science, Oxford, 1997, p18

39 Pomeroy, R. H., 'Shall we cut and reconstruct the perineum for every primipara?' Paper read to American Gynecological Society, 1918. American Journal of Obstetrics and Diseases of Women and Children, Vol. 78, pp211-220

40 DeLee, J. B., 'The Prophylactic Forceps Operation'. Paper read to 45th Annual General Meeting of American Gynecological Society. American Journal of Obstetrics and Gynecology, 1920, pp24-44

41 Quoted in Jacques Maritain, Three Reformers: Luther, Descartes, Rousseau, Scribner, New York, 1950, p184

42 Flint, M., 'Lockmi: An Indian Midwife' in Kay, M. A., op. cit., pp211-219

43 Okley, J., Own or Other Culture, Routledge, London, 1996, pp63-93

44 Maternal Mortality, Ratios and Rates, 3rd ed., WHO, Geneva, 1991

45 Smyke, P., Women and Health, Zed Books, London, 1991

46 Jordan, B., High technology: the case of obstetrics. Paper delivered to World Health Forum, Stockholm, 1987

47 Brady, M. & Shotton, E., 'Midwifery in Sahiwal, Punjab, Pakistan', British Journal of Midwifery, Vol. 3, 7, 1995, pp387-390

48 Ramalingaswami, V., Proven technologies first, World Health Forum, Stockholm, 1987

49 New England Journal of Medicine, 1992, 326: pp1522-1526

50 Special Report on Traditional Midwifery, Suvaguuq, X, 1, Pauktuutit, Inuit Women's Association of Canada, Ottawa, 1995

51 Morewood-Northrop, M., 'Community Birthing Project: Northwest Territories' in Shroff, F. M. (ed) The New Midwifery: Reflections on Renaissance and Regulation, Women's Press, Toronto, 1997, pp343-356

52 Special Report on Traditional Midwifery, Suvsguuk, op. cit.

53 Page, L., The New Midwifery, Cassell, London, 2000

54 Green, J. M., Curtis, P., Price, H. & Renfrew, M. J., Continuing to Care: The organization of midwifery services in the UK: a structural review of the evidence, Midwives Press, Manchester, 1998

Chapter 6

1 Green, J., Coupland, V. & Kitzinger, J., Great Expectations: a prospective study of women's expectations and experiences of childbirth, Child Care and Development Group, Cambridge, 1988

2 McDonald, W. & Davis, J. A., op. cit., p2, p15

3 Chalmers, B., African Birth: Childbirth in cultural transition, Berev, River Club, South Africa 1990, p22

4 Lepori, B., 'Freedom of Movement in Birth Places', Children's Environments, 11 (2), E. & F. N Spon, June 1994, pp81-87

5 Jordan, B., 'The Hut and the Hospital: Information, power and symbolism in the artefacts of birth', Birth 20 (2), 1993, pp36-40

6 Linderman, F., Red Mother, John Day Company, New York, 1932, pp145-147, pp58-61

7 Engelmann, G., Labor Among Primitive Peoples, J. H. Chambers St Louis, 1882, Reprinted AMS Press, New York

8 Notes on Labour in Central Africa, Edinburgh Medical Journal, Vol. XXIX, 1884 pp922-930

9 Englemann, G., op. cit., p15

10 Vincent Priya, J., Birth Traditions and Modern Pregnancy Care, Element, Shaftesbury, 1992, p78

11 Armstrong, P. & Feldman, S., A Midwife's Story, Arbor House, New York, 1986, pp58-61

12 Neumann, Y. S.,'Grandmothers of the Umbilical Cord: traditional midwives in Nicaragua and the birth of a new society', Birth Gazette, 3, 1, (no date), p7

13 Nikodem, W. C., 'Upright versus recumbent position during first stage of labour' in Enkin, M. W., Keirse, M .J. N. C., Renfrew, M. & Neilson, J. P. (eds) Pregnancy and Childbirth Module of Cochrane Database of Systematic Reviews, (updated 24 February 1995); Radkey, A. L., Liston, R. M., Scott, K. E. et al, 'Squatting: preventive medicine in childbirth?' Proceedings of Annual Meeting of Society of Obstetricians and Gynaecologists of Canada, Toronto, 1991, p76

14 Harrison, M., A Woman in Residence, Random House, New York, 1982, p256

15 Englemann, G., op. cit., p29

16 Englemann, G., op. cit., p23

17 Englemann, G., op. cit., p24

18 Englemann, G., op. cit., p43

19 Chalmers, B., op. cit., p19

20 Felkin, R., op. cit.

21 Paciornik, M., 'Arguments Against Episiotomy and In Favor of Squatting for Birth', Birth, Vol. 17, 2, 1990, pp104-105

22 Golay, J., Vedam, S. & Sorger, L., 'The Squatting Position for the Second Stage of Labor: Effects on labor and on maternal and fetal well-being', Birth 20 (2), 1993, pp73-78

23 de Jong, P. R., Johanson, R. B., Baxen, P. et al 'Randomised trial comparing the upright and supine positions for the second stage of labour', British

Journal of Obstetrics and Gynaecology, Vol.104, 5, 1997, pp561-571
24 Engelmann, G., op. cit.
25 Engelmann, G., op. cit., p61-2
26 Chalmers, B., Muggah, H., Samarskaya, M. F. & Tkatchemko, E., 'Women's Experiences of Birth in St Petersburg, Russian Federation, Following a Maternal and Child Health Intervention Program', Birth 25 (2), 1998, pp107-117
27 Cosminsky, S., 'Knowledge and Body Concepts of Guatemalan Midwives' in Kay, M. A., op. cit., pp233-253

Chapter 7
1 Yin-King, L., Holroyd, E., Wong Pui-Yuk, L. et al, 'Hong Kong Chinese women in labour: implications for midwives', The Practising Midwife, Vol. 1 , 11, 1998, pp26-28
2 Neumann, Y. S., 'Grandmothers of the Umbilical Cord: Traditional midwives in Nicaragua', Birth Gazette, Vol. 3, 1, (no date), p7
3 Lederman, C., 'Giving Birth in a Malay Village' in Kay, M. A., op. cit., pp81-100
4 Wertz, R. W. & D. C., op. cit., p78
5 DeLee, J., Obstetrics for Nurses, W. B. Saunders, Philadelphia, 1904, pp107-108
6 Bergstrom, L., Roberts, J., Skillman, I. & Seidel, J., 'You'll Feel Me Touching You Sweetie', Birth 19 (1), 1992, pp10-19
7 Enkin, M. W., 'Commentary: "Do I Do That? Do I Really Do That? Like That?" ', Birth, 19 (1), 1992, pp19-21
8 Jordan, B., Birth in Four Cultures: A cross-cultural investigation of childbirth in Yucatan, Holland, Sweden and the United States, Waveland Press, Prospect Heights, Illinois, 4th Edition 1993, p165
9 Wertz, R. W. & D. C., op. cit., p121
10 Wagner, M. V., Chin, P. V., Peters, C. J., Drexler, B. & Newman, L. A., 'A Comparison of Early and Delayed Induction of Labor with Spontaneous Rupture of Membranes at Term', American Journal of Obstetrics and Gynecology, 74, 1989, pp93-97
11 Perrone, B., Stockel, H. H. & Kreuger, V., Medicine Women, Curanderas, and Women Doctors, Norman: University of Oklahoma Press, 1989
12 Cao-Romero, L., Video, Ticime, Mexico City, 1993
13 Cao-Romero, L., Personal communication, 1994
14 Hulger, M., Together with the Ainu, University of Oklahoma Press, Norman, Oklahoma, p169
15 Hofmeyr, G. J., 'Cephalic version by postural management' in Keirse, M. J. N. C., Renfrew, M. J., Neilson, J. P., & Crowther, C. (eds), Pregnancy and Childbirth Module of Cochrane Database of Systematic Reviews, 1996 (updated 29 February 1996); Zhang, J., Bowes, W. A., Fortney, J. A., 'Efficacy of external cephalic version: a review', American Journal of Obstetrics and Gynecology, Vol. 82, 2, 1993, pp306-312; Shalev, E., Battino, S., Giladi, Y. et al, 'External cephalic version at term - using tocolysis' Acta Obstet Gynecol Scandinavica, Vol. 72, 6, 1993, pp455-457; Flamm, B. L., Fried, M. W., Lonky, N. M. et al, 'External cephalic version after previous cesarean section', American Journal of Obstetrics and Gynecology, Vol. 165, 2, 1991, pp370-372; Fortunato, S. J., Mercer, L. J., Guzick, D. S., 'External cephalic version with tocolysis: factors associated with

success', American Journal of Obstetrics and Gynecology, Vol. 72, 1, 1988, pp59-62; Ferguson, J. E. & Dyson, D. C., 'Intrapartum external cephalic version' in American Journal of Obstetrics and Gynecology, Vol. 152, 3, 1985, pp 297-298
16 Opler, M. E., Childhood and Youth in Jicarilla Apache Society, Frederick Webb Hodge Society Publication Fund, Vol. 5, Los Angeles, 1946
17 McCormack, C., Ethnography of Fertility and Birth, Academic Press, London/New York 1982, pp128-9
18 Perrone, B., Stockel, H. H. & Krueger, V., Medicine Women, Curanderas, and Women Doctors, Norman, University of Oklahoma Press, 1989, p116
19 Fisher, A., 'Reproduction in Truk', Ethnology, 12, 1963, pp526-540
20 The Byrth of Mankind, 1545
21 Encyclopaedia Brittanica, 1797
22 Kitzinger, S., Ourselves as Mothers, Addison-Wesley, Boston, 1994
23 Anon, Medical Knowledge: The Works of the Famous Philosopher, containing his complete Master-Piece and Family Physician, his Experienced Midwife, his book of problems and remarks on physiognomy. To the original work is added, An Essay on Marriage; its duties and enjoyments, J. Smith, London, undated
24 Drew, C. G., 'A Child is Born', She, December 1988
25 Jordan, B., op. cit., p36
26 Spence, 'System of Midwifery', Edinburgh 1784, quoted in George Engelmann, op. cit., p16
27 Engelmann, op. cit., p15
28 Rajadhom, P. A., Some Traditions of the Thai, Thai Inter-Religious Commission for Development and Sathirakoses Nagapradipa Foundation, Bangkok, 1987 p49
29 Smulders, B., Midwifery News, Amsterdam, March 1998. Translated from Dutch
30 Kreiger, D., 'Therapeutic Touch: The Imprimatur of Nursing', American Journal of Nursing 75(5), pp784-787
31 Kitzinger, J. V., 'Counteracting Not Re-enacting, the Violation of Women's Bodies: The Challenge for Prenatal Caregivers', Birth 19, 1992 pp219-227; Kitzinger, J. V., 'The Internal Examination', Practitioner 234, 1990, pp698-700; Kitzinger, J. V., 'Recalling the Pain', Nursing Times 86, 1990, pp38-40; Kitzinger, S., 'Birth and Violence Against Women' in Roberts, H. (ed.) Women's Health Matters, Routledge, London, 1992, pp63-80
32 Van Hoosen, B., 'Scopolamine-Morphine Anaesthesia', New Movement, 42, p121
33 Harrison, M., A Woman in Residence, Random House, New York, 1982, p87
34 Schutz, G. D., 'Mothers Report on Cruelty in Maternity Wards', Ladies' Home Journal 75, 1958, p44
35 Klaus, M. H. & Kennell, J., The Amazing Newborn, Addison Wesley, Reading, Massachusetts, 1985
36 Klaus, M. H. & Kennell, J., op. cit.
37 Elwin, V., 'Conception, Pregnancy and Birth Among the Tribesman of the Maikal Hills', Journal of Royal Asiatic Society of Bengal, Vol 9, 1943
38 Birket-Smith. K., 'An Ethnological Sketch of Rennell Island: A Polynesian Outlier in Melanesia' Det, Congelige Dansk Videnskabelas Selskab, Copenhagen, 1956

39 Boas, F., 'Ethnology of the Kwakiutl', US Bureau of Ethnology 35th Annual Report, 1:1913-14.
40 Rajadhom, P. A., op. cit.
41 Kitzinger, S., 'The Social Context of Birth: Some Comparisons between Childbirth in Jamaica and Britain' in McCormack, C. (ed.) Ethnography of Fertility and Birth, Academic Press, London/New York, 1982, p183
42 Cosminsky, S., 'Knowledge and Body Concepts of Guatemalan Midwives' in Kay, M. A., op. cit., pp 244-246
43 Richardson Hanks, J., 'Maternity and its Ritual' in Bangchan, South East Asian Programme Department, Asian studies, Cornell University, 1963
44 Coughlin, R. J., 'Pregnancy and Birth in the Ainu', 'South East Asian Customs', New Connecticut Human Relations Press, 1965

Chapter 8
1 Vincent, P., 'Traditions of Breastfeeding in Zimbabwe', Newsletter of Birth Traditions Survival Bank, Department of Midwifery Studies, University of Central Lancashire, Preston, Vol. 2, 1993, pp3-7
2 Awang Hasmadi Aswang Mois, op.cit
3 Read, M., Children of Their Fathers, Irvington, 1982
4 Pillsbury, B., 'Doing the Month: Confinement and Convalescence of Chinese Women After Childbirth' in Kay, M. A., op. cit., p127
5 Pillsbury, B., op. cit., p140
6 Jordan, B., op. cit., pp42-44
7 Bartels, L., Birth Songs of the Macha Galla, Ethnology, Vol 8, 1969, pp406-422
8 Minturn, L. & Lambert, W. W., Mothers of Six Cultures, John Wiley and Sons, New York, 1964, p227
9 Pillsbury, B., op. cit., pp119-146
10 Fildes, V., 'The Culture and Biology of Breastfeeding: An Historical View of Western Europe' in Stuart-Macadam, P. & Dettwyler, K. A. (eds) Breastfeeding: Biocultural Perspectives, Aldine De Gruyter, New York, pp101-126
11 Kitzinger, S., 'Commentary' in Stuart-Macadam, P. & Dettwyler, K. A. (eds), op. cit., pp385-394
12 Kitzinger, S., 'Birth and Violence Against Women' in Roberts, H. (ed.), Women's Health Matters, Routledge, London, 1992
13 Chalmers, B., 'Changing Childbirth in Eastern Europe' in Davis-Floyd, R. & Sargent, C. F., Childbirth and Authoritative Knowledge, University of California Press, Berkeley, 1997, pp263-283
14 Konner, M., Childhood: A Multicultural View, Little Brown, Boston, 1991, p62, p196
15 Kitzinger, S., The Crying Baby, Penguin, Harmondsworth, 1990
16 Minturn, L. & Lambert, W. W., op. cit., pp27-8, p222
17 Henderson, L., Kitzinger, J. & Green, J., Representing infant feeding: a content analysis of British media portrayals of bottle feeding and breastfeeding, British Medical Journal, in press, 2000
18 Wilson, A., op. cit.
19 Lancet, Vol. 353, 1999, p1152
20 British Medical Journal, 318, 1999, p1086

Index